I0096791

Harmonious Hormones

= Health

Unlock the Symphony within Your Body

Shania Seeber

Copyright © Shania Seeber 2025

All Rights Reserved

No part of this publication may be reproduced, distributed, or transmitted in any form or by any means, including photocopying, recording, or other electronic or mechanical methods, without the author's prior written permission, except in the case of brief quotations embodied in critical reviews and certain other non-commercial uses permitted by copyright law. For permission requests, please get in touch with the author.

CONTENT

Dedication

This book is dedicated to everyone who has hormones and is alive on planet earth! We are so overwhelmed in our modern world and there is so much biased misinformation online that I hope that this book is impartial and acts as the guide you need.

It is also dedicated to all the moms who trusted me to help them make incredibly amazing human beings. Your babies inspired me to help more women create healthy people and hopefully improve the worlds health one family at a time!

Acknowledgments

I acknowledge all the people who have taught me what I know, either through teaching or mentoring or allowing me to experience their journey with them. Thank you!

About the Author

Dr Shania Seeber's journey to figuring out her own root cause of health started at an early age and developed into a career in complementary alternative medicine, working predominantly in integrative clinics that focussed on longevity and hormones.

She relocated to the United Kingdom in 2016 and has continued to guide patients and educate doctors in the UK on lifestyle medicine. In this book, she offers her personal, practical insights on how to keep your hormones harmonious and happy, so that your body can heal itself the way it is supposed to.

She has written this as a guide for you and it is your formula for harmonious and healthy hormones in the modern world.

Introduction

This book is a companion to my first book "Bad stuff out + Good stuff in = HEALTH" and dives deeper into the effect of bad stuff and good stuff on your hormones. I gained this knowledge through my years of working in integrative practices and I have written this book to help YOU to understand your hormones. How they adjust through a day, a month or a stage of life and the influence you can have on them. Things we should probably be taught to do when we are younger!

We have much more control over our hormones that we are taught. We can affect them through how we manage stress, how we prioritise sleep, by the foods we choose to eat and even the type of exercise we do in the various stages of our lives. If we manage our toxic burden and feed ourselves good nutrients and good relationships, then the symphony that is our hormones, will always play in tune.

Any symptoms associated with a hormonal imbalance, is a message from your body to take note that you need to pay more attention to your day-to-day life.

Through this book, I hope to empower you to understand how you can influence your own health and feel like the best version of yourself. To live not only a long life, but a happy and healthy one.

My aim is to simplify a fairly complex topic, to give you the basics you need to maintain your health and the knowledge of when you should seek medical advice. This book does not take the place of medical advice, it is merely giving you some basic knowledge to empower you to either make the changes you need to make to improve your hormone balance or seek the right medical advice.

I have included both men and women. Men are so often overlooked in the mainstream, but are often seeking help for their, less obvious, hormonal imbalances. I have also included Puberty, as so few books cover this important life stage and our young people need help as well! I hope this book helps you and your family!

Be well,

Dr Shania

Chapter 1

The Symphony of Hormones:

What They Are and How They Shape Your Health

Imagine your body as a grand orchestra. Each instrument plays a vital role, and together, they create a beautiful symphony. But what if one instrument is out of tune? The whole performance could be thrown off balance. In your body, hormones are like the musicians in this orchestra, each one has a specific part to play in keeping you healthy and functioning well.

Understanding hormones is key to understanding how your body works and how you can keep it harmonious and happy.

What Are Hormones?

Hormones are tiny chemical messengers that travel through your bloodstream, carrying instructions from one part of your body to another. These messages tell your cells what to do, when to do it, and how much of something to make. They are produced by glands in the endocrine system, a network of glands that includes the thyroid, adrenal glands, pancreas, ovaries, and testes, among others. Each gland produces different hormones, and each hormone has a unique role in the body.

Think of hormones as the messages your body sends to keep everything running smoothly. Just like you might text a friend to remind them about dinner plans, your body sends out hormones to remind cells to do their jobs, whether it's regulating your temperature, your mood, controlling your appetite, or helping you sleep.

Sounds easy enough, but the symphony changes its tune throughout the day, month and through your life stages, starting at Puberty, then adjusting through the fertile, child bearing years, then through the change of Menopause in women and Andropause in men.

The body is also kept in balance by the nervous system which uses neurotransmitters. Neurotransmitters and hormones are both chemical messengers that work together to help the body communicate and function, but they work in different ways and places. Here's an easy way to think about their differences:

1. Where They Work:

- **Neurotransmitters** are like the body's "instant messengers." They work **in the brain and nervous system**, passing messages between nerve cells (neurons). Think of it like a quick text message; fast and direct.

4

- **Hormones**, on the other hand, are more like mail. They are released into the **bloodstream** and travel to different parts of the body to deliver messages. This process is slower but has a wider reach.

2. Speed:

- **Neurotransmitters** act very quickly; almost instantly, because their job is to keep brain activity, movement, and emotions in check in real-time.

- **Hormones** take more time to have an effect since they must travel through the blood. Their actions are usually longer-lasting, helping with things like growth, metabolism, or mood over hours or days.

3. Specificity:

- **Neurotransmitters** are specific to the nervous system, so they mostly affect processes like mood, memory, sleep, and learning.

- **Hormones** can affect many organs and systems at once, regulating things like growth, energy, or reproduction.

4. Examples:

- A common **neurotransmitter** is **serotonin**, which helps regulate mood and happiness.

- A well-known **hormone** is **insulin**, which helps control blood sugar levels.
- But then there are certain things like **adrenaline**, that acts as both a neurotransmitter and a hormone, to keep to safe from harmful, stressful situations!

In short, neurotransmitters are fast messengers within the nervous system, while hormones take their time, delivering messages throughout the entire body. Both are essential for keeping everything in balance! The focus of this book will be specifically on the hormones and the endocrine system.

Understanding the main hormones and how you can assess and influence them, can make each stage much more harmonious! Let's start with some basics. Starting with Homeostasis.

Homeostasis: Keeping everything in Balance

Homeostasis is your body's way of keeping everything just right, like a special thermostat inside you. Just like how a thermostat in your house keeps the temperature not too hot or too cold, your body has a thermostat that keeps things like your temperature, sugar levels, stress and energy levels balanced.

For example, if you get too hot, your body helps you cool down by sweating. If you're too cold, it makes you shiver to warm up. If you eat a lot of sugar, your body adjusts to use that sugar for energy or store it as fat. Homeostasis is this superhero's job; keeping everything in your body balanced and working perfectly, so you can live your best life, no matter what life stage you are in!

Homeostasis is regulated by several systems in your body, all working together to keep things balanced. The main regulators of homeostasis include:

1. **The Endocrine System:** This system uses hormones, which are like chemical messengers, to control slower, longer-lasting changes. For instance, when your blood sugar is too high, your pancreas releases insulin to help bring it down. This is the system we will focus on in this book, but it is still good to be aware of the others.

2. **The Nervous System:** Your brain and nerves send signals throughout your body to make quick changes. For example, if you touch something hot, your brain tells your muscles to pull your hand away immediately. The main players in your brain are called the Hypothalamus (that's a part of the brain) and the Pituitary gland (a part of the endocrine system in the brain). They are constantly monitoring you and communicating with each other to balance anything that goes out of balance.

Working together, they are the conductors of the orchestra.

3. **The Respiratory System:** Your lungs help maintain the right balance of oxygen and carbon dioxide in your blood by controlling your breathing rate.

4. **The Circulatory System:** Your heart and blood vessels help keep your body temperature stable by moving warm blood to cool areas and vice versa.

5. **The Excretory System:** Your kidneys help balance the amount of water and salt in your body by filtering your blood and making urine. Your liver filters toxins into bile.

Feedback Loops: These are like the body's check-and-balance system. When something is out of balance, feedback loops work to bring it back to normal. There are two types:

- **Negative Feedback Loops:** These reverse a change in the body. For example, if your body gets too hot, it triggers sweating to cool down.

- **Positive Feedback Loops:** These enhance a change. For example, during childbirth, contractions increase through positive feedback until the baby is born.

The good news is that your body knows how to monitor and balance you. It does so constantly! Together, these systems work constantly to keep your body's environment stable, no matter what's happening around you.

The Quick Intro to the Role of Hormones in Your Body

Hormones affect almost every process in your body, from growth and development to metabolism, mood, and reproduction. Let's break down some of the key hormones and their roles:

1. **Insulin: The Blood Sugar Regulator** Insulin is produced by the pancreas and helps control your blood sugar levels. After you eat, insulin signals your cells to take in glucose (sugar) from your bloodstream for energy or storage. If your body doesn't produce enough insulin, that is called type 1 diabetes, which is an autoimmune disease that needs daily insulin to manage it. If your cells don't respond to insulin properly, this is called Insulin resistance or metabolic syndrome and can lead to Type 2 diabetes, which can be reversed or managed through diet and lifestyle changes.

2. **Thyroid Hormones: The Metabolism Managers** The thyroid gland, located in your neck, produces hormones like thyroxine (T4) and triiodothyronine (T3), which regulate your metabolism, which is the rate at which your body burns calories and produces energy. If your

thyroid is underactive (hypothyroidism), you might feel sluggish and gain weight. If it's overactive (hyperthyroidism), you could experience weight loss, anxiety, and a rapid heartbeat.

3. **Cortisol: The Stress Hormone** Cortisol is produced by the adrenal glands, which sit atop your kidneys. It's often called the "stress hormone" because it helps your body respond to stress by increasing blood sugar levels and suppressing non-essential functions, like digestion, during a crisis. While cortisol is essential in small amounts, chronic stress can lead to consistently high cortisol levels, which can disrupt sleep, weaken the immune system, and contribute to weight gain. There are other "stress" hormones and these are discussed in detail in the chapter on the adrenal glands.

4. **Oestrogen and Testosterone: The Sex Hormones** Oestrogen and testosterone are the primary sex hormones. Oestrogen is more dominant in women, and it plays a crucial role in regulating the menstrual cycle, maintaining pregnancy, and supporting bone health. Testosterone, more prevalent in men, is essential for muscle mass, bone density, and sex drive. Both hormones are present in men and women, just in

different amounts, and they influence everything from mood to energy levels. There are more hormones covered under "sex hormones" and will be covered in the chapters related to them, because although they are the same hormones, they have different roles in men and women.

5. **Melatonin: The Sleep Regulator** Produced by the pineal gland in the brain, melatonin helps control your sleep-wake cycle. Levels of melatonin rise in the evening, signalling to your body that it's time to sleep, and fall in the morning as you wake up. Disruptions to your melatonin production, like those caused by too much screen time before bed, can lead to sleep problems. Melatonin has many other functions in the body other than just sleep. It is a powerful anti oxidant. Melatonin also plays a role in the regulation of energy metabolism and glucose homeostasis. It will be discussed in the Stress hormones chapter as it has an ebb and flow relationship with cortisol.

How Hormones Work Together

Just like the instruments in an orchestra need to be in tune with each other, hormones need to work in balance to keep your body healthy. When they're out of balance, it can lead to various health issues. For example, if cortisol levels are too high for too long, it can interfere with insulin's ability to regulate blood sugar, increasing the risk of diabetes. Similarly, imbalances in the stress and sex hormones can influence the thyroid hormones which will then affect metabolism, mood, and energy levels.

Functional medicine looks at hormones as part of a larger, interconnected system. Rather than treating symptoms in isolation, functional medicine aims to understand how different hormones interact and influence each other. This approach helps in identifying the root cause of hormonal imbalances (stress, toxins, etc.) and developing personalised strategies to restore balance.

The Impact of Lifestyle on Hormones

Your lifestyle plays a significant role in how well your hormones function. Factors like diet, exercise, sleep, and stress management can all influence hormone levels. For example:

- Diet: A diet high in sugar and processed foods can cause spikes in insulin, leading to insulin resistance over time. On the other hand, a diet rich in whole foods, healthy fats, and proteins can support stable blood sugar levels and balanced hormone production. Your diet can also influence inflammation, oxidative stress and even support your detox pathways. The food you choose acts either as a positive message and support to your hormones, or can wreak havoc, so choose wisely.

- Exercise: Regular physical activity helps regulate hormones like insulin, cortisol, and growth hormone. It also promotes the production of endorphins, which are natural mood lifters.

- Sleep: Poor sleep can disrupt the production of hormones like melatonin, cortisol, and insulin. Prioritising good sleep hygiene is essential for maintaining hormonal balance. Aim for 8 hours good sleep a night!

- Stress Management: Chronic stress keeps cortisol levels elevated, which can lead to a cascade of other hormonal imbalances. If the stress is sustained over a long period of time, cortisol levels then drop and this leads to symptoms such as fatigue and salt cravings. Techniques like meditation, deep breathing, and regular exercise can help manage stress and support healthy cortisol levels. There are also nutrients and supplements that can help and these will be covered in detail in the chapter on stress.

Taking Control of Your Hormonal Health

Understanding hormones gives you the power to take control of your health. By paying attention to your body's signals and making lifestyle choices that support hormonal balance, you can optimise your overall well-being.

If you suspect you have a hormonal imbalance, it's important to work with a healthcare provider who can evaluate your symptoms and recommend appropriate testing and work on the root cause of the symptoms. Functional medicine practitioners are particularly skilled at looking at the whole picture and helping you find the root cause of your symptoms.

Remember, your hormones are not just isolated chemicals, they're part of a complex and interconnected system that influences every aspect of your health. By keeping them in balance, you're helping to ensure that your body's symphony plays on in perfect harmony.

Chapter 2

The Symphony of Hormones: Navigating Stress, Environmental Toxins & Gut Health

As described in the previous chapter, hormones are the body's chemical messengers, orchestrating a delicate symphony that regulates nearly every function within us including mood, metabolism, energy levels, sleep, growth, reproduction, and more. This symphony requires precise timing and balance, with each hormone playing its part to ensure the body's systems operate harmoniously. However, like any finely tuned instrument, hormones can be disrupted by external influences, particularly stress and environmental toxins.

In this chapter, we'll explore how stress and exposure to environmental toxins like heavy metals, the mycotoxin Zearalenone, and persistent pollutants such as Bisphenol-A (BPA), disrupt the hormonal balance, leading to various health issues. We'll also discuss strategies to protect your hormonal health by minimising exposure to these harmful substances and managing stress effectively.

The Impact of Stress on Hormones

Stress is an unavoidable part of life, but chronic stress can be particularly harmful to hormonal balance. When the body perceives a threat, whether real or imagined, it activates the "fight or flight" response, leading to the release of cortisol and adrenaline/epinephrine. I will refer to adrenaline in the book, but it is also known as epinephrine in some parts of the world

Adrenaline and cortisol are the two key hormones that help the body manage stress, but they work in different ways to prepare and protect us when we face challenges. Here's how they handle stress:

1. Adrenaline: The Immediate Response ("Fight or Flight")

- When you experience a stressful situation (like a sudden danger or shock), **adrenaline** is released almost instantly from the adrenal glands, which sit on top of your kidneys.

- Adrenaline gives you a **quick burst of energy** by:
    - Increasing your heart rate and blood pressure, sending more oxygen and blood to your muscles.
    - Dilating your airways so you can take in more oxygen.
    - Sharpening your focus and reactions, making you more alert.

- This "fight or flight" response is meant to help you either confront the stressor or escape from it as fast as possible.

- For example, if you were in a dangerous situation, adrenaline would help you move quickly and respond faster.

2. Cortisol: The Longer-Term Stress Manager

- **Cortisol**, also produced by the adrenal glands, kicks in when stress is more prolonged or chronic. While adrenaline deals with the immediate threat, cortisol is there for the long haul.

- Cortisol helps by:
    - Keeping your **energy levels** up by releasing glucose (sugar) into your bloodstream.
    - Suppressing functions that aren't essential in the moment (like digestion or reproduction) to conserve energy.
    - **Regulating inflammation** and maintaining a balanced immune response to prevent damage from prolonged stress.

- If stress continues over a long period, cortisol keeps your body alert and ready, but too much can lead to problems like fatigue, weight gain, or a weakened immune system.

In Summary:

- **Adrenaline** is your body's **emergency alarm**—it gives you the immediate boost needed to deal with a sudden stressor.

- **Cortisol** is more of a **stress manager**—it helps sustain your energy and focus over longer periods of stress but needs to be balanced to avoid health issues.

Together, they create a powerful system that helps you survive and adapt to stressful situations, but chronic stress can disrupt the balance, leading to health problems.

Let's Look Deeper How Stress Affects Us

- **Short-Term vs. Chronic Stress**: In the short term, cortisol helps the body cope with stress by increasing energy production, suppressing non-essential functions, and enhancing the immune response. However, chronic stress leads to prolonged cortisol production, which can cause a host of issues, including weight gain, insomnia, anxiety, depression, and weakened immune function.

- **Disrupting Other Hormones:** Chronic cortisol elevation disrupts the balance of other hormones. For example, high cortisol levels can suppress the production of thyroid hormones, leading to hypothyroidism symptoms like fatigue, weight gain, and depression. Cortisol can also inhibit progesterone production, contributing to oestrogen dominance and related conditions like PMS, fibroids, and endometriosis.

- **Effect on Reproductive Hormones:** Chronic stress can disrupt the menstrual cycle, leading to irregular periods or amenorrhea (absence of menstruation). It can also reduce libido and impair fertility in both men and women.

- **Impact on Blood Sugar and Insulin:** Cortisol raises blood sugar levels by promoting gluconeogenesis (the production of glucose from non-carbohydrate sources). Over time, this can lead to insulin resistance, weight gain, and an increased risk of type 2 diabetes.

Strategies for Managing Stress

- **Removing the Stressor:** This may sound easier than it is to do. If you can't take yourself out of the stressful environment, then another thing to try is to adjust the way you respond to it. This is hard but is very effective. You actually do have a choice on how you allow things to stress you and changing the way you respond, by choosing to walk away and be quiet instead of reacting, or taking a break in nature before reacting or actively choosing peace over stress can have an effect on your stress hormones. It takes patience and practice!

- **Mindfulness and Relaxation Techniques:** Practices like meditation, deep breathing, and mindful exercise, can help lower cortisol levels and promote relaxation. Regular practice of these techniques can build resilience to stress.

- **Physical Activity:** Regular exercise helps regulate cortisol levels, improve mood, and enhance overall well-being. Aim for a balance of aerobic exercise, strength training, and flexibility exercises.

- **Adequate Sleep:** Quality sleep is essential for regulating cortisol and other hormones. Create a sleep-friendly environment, maintain a regular sleep schedule, and practice good sleep hygiene.

- **Healthy Diet:** A balanced diet rich in whole foods, healthy fats, and good quality proteins supports hormonal health and helps the body cope with stress. Limiting caffeine and sugar can also help reduce cortisol levels.

Environmental Toxins and Hormonal Disruption

Beyond physical and emotional stress, environmental toxins represent a significant threat to hormonal balance. These substances, often referred to as endocrine disruptors, can mimic, block, or interfere with the body's natural hormones. They are found in various sources, including food, water, air, and consumer products such as skin products and household cleaning products.

Heavy Metals: A Silent Threat

Heavy metals like mercury, lead, and cadmium are pervasive environmental pollutants with known toxic effects on human health. They can accumulate in the body over time, disrupting the endocrine system and leading to various health issues. Even metals that have a function in the body, such as copper and iron, in excess or deficiency, can impact your hormones and should be kept in balance.

- **Mercury:** Found in contaminated fish (worse in fish that eat other fish, like Tuna or swordfish), dental fillings, and industrial emissions, mercury can impair thyroid function, disrupt the menstrual cycle, and contribute to infertility and even chronic pain conditions such as fibromyalgia.

- **Lead:** Historically used in petrol, paints and water pipes, lead exposure can cause developmental issues in children and hormonal imbalances in adults, including disruptions in reproductive hormones and thyroid function. A common symptom of lead toxicity is joint pain.

- **Cadmium:** Found in cigarette smoke, batteries, and contaminated food, cadmium exposure has been linked to kidney damage, bone loss, and disruptions in oestrogen and testosterone levels. It is a known antagonist of zinc, which is important for many life functions including hormones.

Zearalenone: The Fungal Oestrogen

Most mycotoxins are bad things to have in your body. Zearalenone is a mycotoxin produced by certain fungi that contaminate crops like corn and wheat. It mimics oestrogen in the body and can lead to oestrogen dominance-like symptoms, contributing to reproductive issues like PMS, fibroids, and early puberty in girls.

- **Impact on Women's Health:** Zearalenone exposure can exacerbate conditions like endometriosis and fibrocystic breast disease by increasing oestrogen activity in the body.

- **Impact on Men's Health:** Zearalenone will contribute to oestrogenic symptoms like the growth of breast tissue.

- **Food Contamination:** Zearalenone is most commonly found in contaminated grains and grain-based products. Consuming organic, non-GMO foods and properly storing grains can reduce exposure.

Persistent Organic Pollutants: Forever Chemicals

Persistent organic pollutants (POPs) include substances like bisphenol-A (BPA), phthalates, PFAS, dioxins, and PCBs. These chemicals are resistant to environmental degradation and can accumulate in the human body, leading to long-term health effects.

- **Bisphenol-A (BPA):** There is a whole family of Bisphenols, not just A and they are all bad! Commonly found in plastics, food containers, the lining of canned foods, and thermal receipts, BPA is an endocrine disruptor that mimics oestrogen and can contribute to hormone-related conditions such as breast cancer, obesity, and reproductive disorders. This is why it is recommended to avoid plastics, especially heated plastic, which releases the BPA's into your food.

- **Phthalates:** Used as plasticisers in products like cosmetics, toys, and medical devices, phthalates disrupt testosterone and oestrogen production, potentially leading to reproductive issues, developmental problems, and metabolic disorders.

- **PFAS:** PFAS (per- and polyfluoroalkyl substances) are synthetic chemicals known for their resistance to heat, water, and oil, and they are found in various consumer products. These chemicals are persistent in the environment and human body, earning them the nickname "forever chemicals." PFAS have been linked to several health effects, including disruptions to the endocrine (hormonal) system, specifically affecting the thyroid hormones, sex hormones, insulin and even cortisol.

- **Dioxins and PCBs:** These toxic chemicals, produced by industrial processes and found in the environment, can interfere with thyroid function, immune response, and reproductive health.

Mitigating the Impact of Environmental Toxins

- **Reduce Exposure:** Minimise exposure to endocrine disruptors by choosing products labelled BPA-free, avoiding plastic containers for food storage, and choosing organic produce when possible. Read labels and be mindful of products containing phthalates and choose natural alternatives for personal care products.

- **Support Detoxification:** The body has natural detoxification pathways, primarily through the liver, that can be supported by a healthy diet rich in antioxidants, fibre, and hydration. Foods like cruciferous vegetables (broccoli, cauliflower, kale) and herbs like coriander/cilantro and milk thistle can support liver function and the elimination of toxins. Other foods like lemon zest, flaxseeds, rosemary, dandelion tea, rooibos tea, colourful berries and good quality protein can also all add value.

- **Filter Water and Air:** Use high-quality water filters to remove heavy metals and contaminants from drinking and bathing water and consider air purifiers to reduce exposure to airborne pollutants.

- **Safer Food Choices:** Limit consumption of large, predatory fish known to contain higher levels of mercury, such as tuna, shark and swordfish, and choose wild-caught (not farmed), smaller fish, like salmon or sardines. Properly wash and store food to reduce exposure to zearalenone and other contaminants.

The Role of a Healthy Gut:

Although not a part of the external environment, the gut is a part of the body that has direct contact to the foods introduced from the external environment, so much so, that 70% of the immune system is located in it. A healthy gut also plays a vital role in maintaining hormone balance, as the digestive system and hormones are closely interconnected. Here's how a well-functioning gut contributes to hormone balance:

1. Hormone Production and Regulation

- **Serotonin Production:** The gut produces about 90% of the body's serotonin, a neurotransmitter that influences mood, sleep, and appetite. Serotonin also plays a role in regulating other hormones, such as melatonin, which controls sleep-wake cycles.

- **Oestrogen Metabolism:** The gut helps regulate oestrogen levels through the "estrobolome," a collection of gut bacteria that metabolise oestrogen. A healthy gut ensures proper oestrogen breakdown and elimination, preventing excess oestrogen that could lead to hormonal imbalances like PMS or oestrogen dominance. An unhealthy microbiome can make an enzyme called beta glucuronidase, that uncouples oestrogen that has been bound in the liver and moved into the gut to be removed. That uncoupling releases the oestrogen and it is reabsorbed back into the body contributing to an excess of oestrogen.

2. Detoxification and Elimination

- **Excretion of Hormones:** The liver processes and detoxifies hormones like oestrogen, cortisol, and thyroid hormones, which are then excreted through the bile into the intestines. A healthy gut ensures these hormones are properly eliminated from the body. If gut health is compromised (e.g., with dysbiosis or constipation), these hormones can be reabsorbed, leading to imbalances.

3. Gut Microbiome and Hormonal Communication

- **Microbiome Influence:** The gut microbiome, the community of bacteria in the digestive tract, communicates with the endocrine system. Healthy gut bacteria support the production and regulation of hormones, while an imbalance in gut bacteria (dysbiosis) can lead to hormonal disruptions.

- **Immune Function:** A healthy gut supports the immune system, which indirectly affects hormone balance. Chronic inflammation, often rooted in poor gut health, can disrupt the delicate balance of hormones, particularly stress hormones like cortisol.

4. Nutrient Absorption

- **Vitamin and Mineral Absorption:** The gut is responsible for absorbing nutrients from food, including vitamins and minerals essential for hormone production and balance. For example, vitamins B6, B12, and folate are critical for hormone regulation, and these nutrients must be absorbed efficiently in the gut.

- **Fatty Acids:** Healthy fats are crucial for hormone production, particularly sex hormones like oestrogen, progesterone, and testosterone. A healthy gut ensures the proper digestion and absorption of these fats.

5. Stress Response and the Gut-Brain Axis

- **Gut-Brain Connection:** The gut and brain communicate through the gut-brain axis, influencing stress hormones like cortisol. A healthy gut can help regulate stress responses, preventing cortisol imbalances that can affect other hormones.

- **Stress and stomach acid:** Stomach acid kills bad bugs before they enter the rest of the gut, but also digests proteins. Unfortunately, not chewing your food well, eating too fast, eating when stressed and having certain nutrient deficiencies, can lead to your stomach acid not being strong enough to do these 2 vital functions.

A healthy gut is essential for hormone balance by supporting hormone production, detoxification, and communication between the gut and endocrine systems. Maintaining gut health through a balanced diet, probiotics, fibre, and stress management can help keep your hormones in harmony, promoting overall well-being.

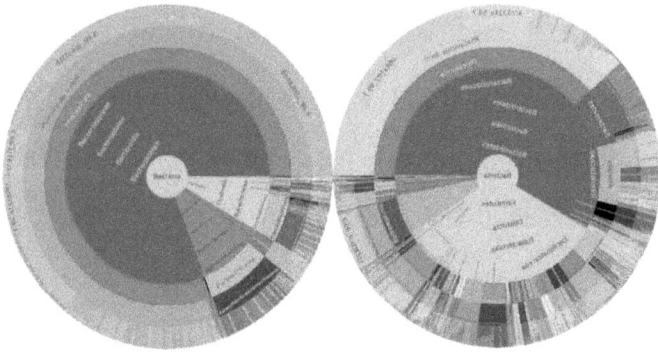

Here we see examples of an unhealthy microbiome on the left and a healthy microbiome on the right, where the results are more colourful and balanced.

Conclusion: Harmonising Your Hormonal Symphony

Your hormones play a vital role in maintaining your health and well-being. The balance of this intricate hormonal symphony can be easily disrupted by stress and environmental toxins, leading to a cascade of health issues. However, by understanding these risks and taking proactive steps to manage stress and reduce exposure to harmful substances, you can protect your hormonal health and support overall well-being.

Incorporating stress management techniques, adopting a clean diet, and making mindful choices about the products you use can help you maintain the harmony of your hormones.

Remember, your body is resilient, and with the right care and attention, you can keep your hormonal symphony in tune, leading to a healthier and more vibrant life.

Chapter 3

Feeding Your Hormones: The Crucial Role of Nutrition in Hormonal Health

We've talked about how hormones are like the musicians in your body's orchestra, each playing a vital role in keeping your health in harmony. We've also discussed the environmental factors that can disrupt this delicate balance. Now, it's time to focus on a powerful tool you have at your disposal to support your hormonal health: Nutrition.

Just as a musician needs a well-tuned instrument and the right sheet music to perform at their best, your hormones need the right nutrients to function optimally. The food you eat is more than just fuel, it's the raw material your body uses to produce and regulate hormones. In this chapter, we'll explore how the different components of your diet; fats, proteins, carbohydrates, vitamins, and minerals, play a crucial role in maintaining hormonal balance.

The Foundation of Hormones: Fats and Proteins

To understand the importance of nutrition for hormonal health, it helps to start with the basics: fats and proteins as they are both the main building blocks of hormones.

Fats: The Building Blocks of Hormones

Fats have often been misunderstood and unfairly vilified, but they are absolutely essential for hormonal health. In fact, many hormones are made from cholesterol, a type of fat that you have probably heard about in relation to heart health, but it is also an essential fat building block for many hormones. Without adequate fat intake, your body can't produce key hormones like oestrogen, testosterone, and cortisol. These hormones are called "steroid" hormones.

There are different types of dietary fats, and not all of them are equally beneficial. Here's what you need to know:

- **Saturated Fats and Cholesterol:** These fats are generally solid when cool and liquid when heated. They are found in foods like butter, eggs, and meat. While saturated fats have been demonised in the past, they play a critical role in hormone production. Cholesterol, in particular, is the precursor to several important hormones, including the sex hormones and adrenal hormones.

- **Monounsaturated Fats:** Found in foods like avocados, olive oil, and nuts, these fats are heart-healthy and support hormone production. They also help maintain cell membranes, which are crucial for hormone receptors to function properly.

- **Polyunsaturated Fats (Omega-3 and Omega-6):** Omega-3 fatty acids, found in flaxseeds, walnuts, grass fed meat and fatty fish like salmon, have anti-inflammatory properties that support hormonal health. Omega-6 fatty acids, found in vegetable oils and seeds, are also essential, but it's important to maintain a balance between omega-3 and omega-6 intake to prevent inflammation, which can disrupt hormones. It is relatively easy to test this balance and adjust your diet according to your specific needs.

- **Trans Fats:** These are the unhealthy fats found in many processed foods. Trans fats can interfere with hormone receptors and disrupt the balance of hormones in the body. Avoiding trans fats is crucial for maintaining hormonal health.

Proteins: The Hormone Building Blocks

Proteins are made up of amino acids, which are the building blocks of many hormones and enzymes in your body. For example, insulin, a hormone that regulates blood sugar, and the thyroid hormones, which are essential for tissue repair and metabolism, are both based on the amino acids from proteins.

When you eat protein-rich foods, your body breaks them down into amino acids, which are then used to produce hormones, repair tissues, and perform countless other functions. Ensuring you get enough high-quality protein in your diet is essential for supporting these processes. It is also important to properly digest and absorb the proteins. This starts with chewing your food well. It is also important that your stomach is acid enough to continue the digestion of the proteins as this digestion ends at the stomach. If you have had lots of stress or are deficient in nutrients such as zinc, your stomach may not reach a pH low enough to break the protein down into amino acids which can then be absorbed. If this is the case, you may benefit from a digestive supplement.

Some excellent sources of protein include:

- **Animal-Based Proteins:** Eggs, poultry, fish, grass fed beef, lamb, and dairy products provide complete proteins, meaning they contain all the essential amino acids your body needs. It is best to support local, regenerative farmers, who ensure their animals are well looked after.

- **Plant-Based Proteins:** As many people are choosing not to eat meat, plant options are their only choice, but meat eaters should also consider getting some protein from these sources as well as they are good for gut health and more. Legumes, nuts, seeds, and soy products like tofu and tempeh are excellent sources of protein for those who follow a plant-based diet. While most plant proteins are not complete on their own, eating a variety of these foods ensures you get all the essential amino acids.

And then there are the Carbohydrates: Energy Source

Carbohydrates (carbs), formed of fibre, starches and sugars, are essential food nutrients, even though some are demonised as being bad, whole carbohydrates do have benefits other than just adding sugar to your body. Your body turns carbs into glucose (blood sugar) to give you the energy you need to function. Complex carbs in fruits, vegetables and whole-grain foods are less likely to spike blood sugar than simple carbs (sugars) and contain other nutrients like minerals and polyphenols, that help your body function better, by reducing inflammation and oxidative stress.

A hormone-supportive diet isn't just about the *quantity* of carbohydrates. It's also important to consider the *quality* of carbohydrates and the timing of when you're eating them throughout the day. Choosing high fibre carbohydrates, such as those found in whole grains, legumes, and colourful vegetables provide the essential nutrients needed to support proper hormone function. Also, the fibre in complex carbohydrates also helps slow the release of carbohydrates into the bloodstream, thus keeping blood sugar more stable. The fibre has the added benefit of being a food source for your microbiome, so remember, you aren't just feeding your own body but also the millions of bugs that keep you healthy from the inside!

The best time to eat carbohydrates to help balance blood sugar depends on several factors, such as your activity level, individual metabolism, and the type of carbs you're consuming. However, here are some general guidelines for optimal timing:

1. Pair Carbs with Protein and Fat

- Instead of eating carbs on their own, it's best to consume them alongside protein and healthy fats. This combination helps **slow down the digestion of carbohydrates**, preventing sudden spikes in blood sugar. For example, having whole-grain toast with avocado and eggs can help keep your blood sugar steady compared to eating toast alone.

2. Spread Carbs Throughout the Day

- To avoid blood sugar highs and lows, it's important to **spread your carb intake throughout the day**. Eating small to moderate portions of carbs at each meal helps maintain a stable blood sugar level rather than causing sudden increases.

- Try to include complex carbs (like whole grains, vegetables, and legumes) with each meal, as they are digested more slowly and have a gentler effect on blood sugar.

3. Eat Carbs Earlier in the Day

- **Morning and lunchtime** are often the best times to consume the majority of your carbohydrates. At these times, your body is typically more insulin-sensitive, meaning it can process carbs more efficiently. A balanced breakfast with protein, fat, and fibre-rich carbs can set you up for more stable energy throughout the day. Cereals on their own are not generally a good breakfast idea!

- A carb-heavy meal late in the evening, however, may cause blood sugar spikes overnight, especially if the carbs are refined (like white bread or pasta).

4. Time Carbs Around Exercise

- If you are physically active, eating **carbohydrates before and after exercise** can help balance blood sugar. Before exercise, carbs provide the energy your muscles need. Afterward, carbs help **replenish glycogen stores** and support recovery.

- For example, a small snack with carbs and protein, like a banana with peanut butter, can be beneficial before a workout, while a post-workout meal that includes complex carbs can help balance your energy afterward. Cold baked baby potatoes are generally considered a healthy option as they contain **Resistant starch** which positively impacts the glycaemic response.

5. Avoid Large Amounts of Simple Carbs in One Sitting

- Foods high in **simple carbohydrates** (like sugary snacks, white bread, and sweets) are quickly broken down and absorbed, causing **rapid spikes in blood sugar**. Instead, opt for **complex carbohydrates** like oats, quinoa, and sweet potatoes, which have a slower, more controlled release of glucose.

The best approach is to eat carbohydrates in **moderation**, paired with protein and fats, and distributed evenly across your meals—especially earlier in the day or around physical activity. This helps keep blood sugar levels more stable and prevents sudden highs and lows. If you want to control your glucose levels, you can consider berberine and chromium supplements.

Essential Nutrients for Hormonal Health

The Minerals: The Spark plugs of Metabolism

Beyond carbohydrates, fats and proteins, certain vitamins and minerals play specific roles in hormone production and regulation. Let's explore some of the key nutrients that are particularly important for keeping your hormones in balance.

Zinc: The Hormone Helper

Zinc is a trace mineral that plays a vital role in hormone production and regulation. It's particularly important for reproductive health, as it supports the production of testosterone in men and helps regulate the menstrual cycle in women. Zinc also plays a role in insulin production and thyroid function. It is also an essential nutrient for the stomach.

Foods rich in zinc include oysters, beef, pumpkin seeds, lentils, and chickpeas. If you're not getting enough zinc in your diet, it can lead to hormonal imbalances, weakened immune function, and impaired wound healing and you may need to consider a supplement.

Copper: The Balancer

Copper works closely with zinc to maintain a balance of hormones in the body. It's involved in the production of energy, the formation of connective tissue, and the regulation of neurotransmitters that affect mood. However, it's important to maintain a proper balance between zinc and copper, as too much of one can deplete the other. Copper really needs to be kept in balance, too much or too little will cause health issues.

Good dietary sources of copper include liver, shellfish, nuts, seeds, whole grains, and dark leafy greens. Maintaining the right balance of copper and zinc is crucial for preventing conditions like anaemia, cardiovascular disease, and hormonal imbalances.

Copper and oestrogen are intricately related. Copper toxicity and excess copper levels causes the body to hold onto oestrogen in the body and prevent its detoxification, and having excess oestrogen levels and poor oestrogen detoxification causes the body to hold onto copper. This is more commonly seen these days, ever since the pill was invented in the 1950's. The original pill had a very high dose of oestrogen which caused women using it to store copper. This copper, unless it was actively removed, was transferred to the baby girl that woman gave birth to and then that was passed on to the next generation. This has continued for a few generations; each one being passed on a burden of extra copper. I highly recommend assessing copper in any condition related to oestrogen.

Iron: The Energy Enabler

Iron is essential for the production of haemoglobin, the protein in red blood cells that carries oxygen throughout your body. But iron also plays a role in thyroid function and hormone production. Without enough iron, you might experience fatigue, mood swings, and other symptoms of hormonal imbalance.

Iron is found in two forms in food: haem iron (found in animal products like red meat, poultry, and fish) and non- haem iron (found in plant-based foods like lentils, beans, and spinach). Haem iron is more easily absorbed by the body, but pairing non-haem iron sources with vitamin C-rich foods (like citrus fruits or bell peppers) can enhance absorption.

Selenium: The Thyroid Protector

Selenium is a powerful antioxidant that plays a critical role in thyroid health. The thyroid gland uses selenium to produce thyroid hormones and to protect itself from oxidative damage. Selenium is also involved in the conversion of the thyroid hormone T4 (inactive) into T3 (active), which regulates metabolism.

Brazil nuts used to be one of the richest sources of selenium, with just one or two nuts a day providing your daily requirement, however, the trees are now being grown in areas that have been depleted of their selenium, so Brazil nuts are not always as rich in selenium as they used to be. Other good sources include seafood, eggs, and sunflower seeds.

Iodine: Thyroid Essential

Necessary to produce thyroid hormones. The body also needs thyroid hormones for proper bone and brain development during pregnancy and infancy. It can also help breast tissue that has become fibrocystic.

Iodine is found in iodised salt, seaweed, and dairy products.

Magnesium: The Stress Reliever

Magnesium is often referred to as the "relaxation mineral" because of its calming effects on the nervous system. It helps regulate cortisol levels, promoting a balanced stress response. Magnesium also plays a role in the production of sex hormones like oestrogen and testosterone, as well as in the activation of vitamin D, which supports hormone production. It is also involved in blood sugar regulation; in fact it has 100's of known functions in the human body. Most people are deficient in magnesium and require some form of supplement.

You can find magnesium in foods like dark leafy greens, nuts, seeds, whole grains, and dark chocolate. If you're not getting enough magnesium, you might experience symptoms like anxiety, muscle cramps, constipation or difficulty sleeping, all of which can be linked to hormonal imbalances.

Vitamins: The Hormone Supporters

Vitamins are essential for overall health, and certain vitamins play key roles in hormone production and regulation. Let's look at some of the most important ones for hormonal balance.

Vitamin D: The Sunshine Hormone

Vitamin D is unique because it functions more like a hormone than a vitamin. Your body produces vitamin D when your skin is exposed to sunlight, and it plays a crucial role in calcium absorption, immune function, and the production of sex hormones. Vitamin D is also involved in regulating dopamine, insulin and supporting thyroid function.

Many people are deficient in vitamin D, especially during the winter months or if they spend little time outdoors. Foods like fatty fish, egg yolks, and fortified dairy products can help boost your vitamin D levels, but sunlight remains the most effective source.

A blood test can determine if you need a supplement to reach optimal levels. If you supplement vitamin D, consider adding vitamin K which can guide the vitamin D into the bones. While vitamin D3 helps your body absorb more calcium, vitamin K2 helps your body transport it to your bones and teeth rather than letting it sit in your arteries and other soft tissues in your body. This not only helps to promote bone health, but it also helps to keep your heart healthy as well.

Vitamin B5: Stress Manager

Vitamin B5, also known as pantothenic acid, plays a crucial role in supporting the adrenal glands, which are responsible for producing adrenal hormones like cortisol and adrenaline.

As you now know, cortisol is a hormone that helps your body respond to stress. Vitamin B5 is involved in making cortisol, helping the adrenal glands produce enough of this hormone when needed. Without sufficient vitamin B5, cortisol production can be impaired, making it harder for the body to manage stress effectively.

Vitamin B6: The Hormone Regulator

Vitamin B6 is essential for the production of neurotransmitters like serotonin and dopamine, which influence mood and stress levels. It also plays a role in regulating oestrogen and progesterone, making it particularly important for women's health and is often prescribed along with magnesium to improve many of the symptoms seen in PMS.

Foods rich in vitamin B6 include poultry, fish, potatoes, bananas, and chickpeas. Adequate B6 intake can help reduce symptoms of PMS, improve mood, and support overall hormonal balance.

Vitamin B9 (Folate): Methylation Manager

Vitamin B9, also known as folate or folic acid (in its synthetic form, which may not be good for people with the MTHFR TT variant), plays a critical role in the process of methylation, which is essential for overall health. Methylation is a biochemical process that involves adding a methyl group (one carbon and three hydrogen atoms) to various molecules in the body that changes that molecules shape and function in the body.

This process is vital for numerous bodily functions, including producing and repairing DNA, which is necessary for cell division and growth. Proper methylation ensures that DNA is replicated accurately, helping to prevent mutations that could lead to health issues like heart disease, depression and cancer.

Vitamin B9 is essential for gene expression, neurotransmitter production, detoxification, and cardiovascular health. Proper folate intake is crucial for maintaining these vital functions and overall well-being.

Vitamin B12: The Energy Booster

Vitamin B12 is crucial for energy production, nervous system function, and the formation of red blood cells. It also supports thyroid function and helps maintain healthy levels of homocysteine; an amino acid linked to cardiovascular health.

Vitamin B12 is found naturally in animal products like meat, fish, eggs, and dairy. For vegetarians and vegans, fortified foods or supplements are often necessary to ensure adequate intake.

Vitamin C: The Antioxidant Powerhouse

Vitamin C is a powerful antioxidant that supports adrenal gland function and the production of stress hormones like cortisol. It also helps protect other hormones from oxidative damage and supports the immune system. Vitamin C also helps with progesterone production.

Citrus fruits, berries, bell peppers, and broccoli are all excellent sources of vitamin C. Including these foods in your diet can help your body manage stress and maintain hormonal balance.

Polyphenols: The Protective Colours

There are many polyphenols! They are found in foods like green tea, berries, and dark chocolate. Polyphenols reduce oxidative stress and inflammation, which can impact hormone balance.

Phytoestrogens: Plant based Oestrogen

Isoflavones: Found in soy products like tofu and tempeh, isoflavones are plant compounds that can mimic or modulate oestrogen in the body, helping balance hormone levels in both men and women.

Soluble and Insoluble Fiber: Microbiome Magic

Found in fruits, vegetables, whole grains, and legumes, fibre is crucial for maintaining a healthy gut and microbiome, which in turn supports hormone metabolism and the elimination of excess hormones like oestrogen.

Adaptogens (these will be discussed in detail in Chapter 5)

Maca Root: A plant native to Peru, maca is believed to support energy levels, libido, and hormone balance, particularly in women.

Ashwagandha: Used in Ayurvedic medicine, this herb helps regulate cortisol levels and supports overall hormonal balance, particularly during stress.

Nourishing Your Hormones for Optimal Health

Your hormones rely on the nutrients you provide through your diet to function properly. By prioritising a balanced diet rich in healthy fats, high-quality proteins, healthy complex carbohydrates and essential vitamins and minerals, you're giving your body the tools it needs to produce and regulate hormones effectively.

Conclusion:

In functional medicine, we emphasise the importance of a whole-foods-based diet to support overall health. This approach not only helps maintain hormonal balance but also reduces the risk of chronic diseases, improves energy levels, and enhances your quality of life.

Remember, the choices you make at every meal have a direct impact on your hormonal health. By nourishing your body with the right nutrients, you can help ensure that your hormones remain in harmony, allowing your body's orchestra to play a beautiful, balanced symphony every day.

Chapter 4

The Thyroid: Your Body's Metabolic Maestro

The thyroid gland is often referred to as the "master controller" of your metabolism. Located at the base of your neck, this small, butterfly-shaped gland plays an enormous role in regulating your body's energy production, temperature, and overall metabolic rate. In this chapter, we'll dive deeper into the key thyroid hormones - TSH, T3, T4, and reverse T3 - and explore what impacts their function.

Thyroid dysfunction is notoriously underdiagnosed, with as many 60% of people with thyroid dysfunction are unaware of it. Statistics show that women are seven times more likely than men to develop thyroid issues in their lifetime, but especially during peri-menopause, when all hormones start fluctuating.

Understanding Thyroid Hormones: TSH, T3, T4, and rT3

The thyroid gland produces hormones that affect almost every cell in your body. The primary hormones involved in this process are:

- Thyroid-Stimulating Hormone (TSH)
- Triiodothyronine (T3)
- Thyroxine (T4)
- Reverse Triiodothyronine (rT3).

Let's break down what each of these hormones does and how they work together to keep your metabolism in check.

TSH: The Thyroid Manager

TSH, or Thyroid-Stimulating Hormone, is produced by the pituitary gland in the brain. Think of TSH as the manager that oversees the thyroid gland's operations. Its primary job is to regulate the production T4 by signalling the thyroid to produce more or less of the hormone depending on the body's needs.

When TSH levels are high, it's usually a sign that the thyroid isn't producing enough thyroid hormones (a condition known as hypothyroidism). Conversely, low TSH levels typically indicate that the thyroid is overproducing hormones (a condition known as hyperthyroidism). Monitoring TSH levels is often the first step in assessing thyroid health. But it isn't the only hormone that should be tested and in most conventional cases, it is the only test that is done!

The normal reference range for thyroid-stimulating hormone (TSH) levels is typically between 0.45 and 4.5 milliunits per litre (mU/L). However, the normal range can vary depending on a number of factors, including:

- Age: Some labs use a higher normal range for older people, as high as 7 µU/mL.

- Pregnancy: The normal range for TSH is different for pregnant women.

- Laboratory: Different labs may use different measurements or test different samples, so normal ranges may vary slightly.

- Medications: Some medications and supplements (like biotin) can modify thyroid hormone metabolism.

TSH levels can also vary during the day, so it's best to have the test early in the morning. Also, note that even if you fall within the reference range, if your results are trending higher in that range, that may indicate sub optimal thyroid function, especially if you have symptoms.

T4: The Inactive Precursor

Thyroxine, or T4, is the primary hormone produced by the thyroid gland, making up about 80% of the thyroid hormones in your body. However, T4 is relatively inactive on its own. It serves as a precursor to the more active T3 hormone. T4 is like the raw material that needs to be converted into something more functional to have a significant impact on your metabolism.

Using the nutrients iron and selenium, your liver and other tissues convert T4 into the active T3, which then exerts its effects on the body's cells. This conversion process is crucial for maintaining energy levels, regulating metabolism, and supporting overall health.

T4 can be tested in both its free form and Total T4. Total T4 includes both free T4 and the T4 that is bound to a protein. It is an indicator of the thyroid glands ability to synthesise, process and release T4 into the bloodstream.

T3: The Active Hormone

Triiodothyronine, or T3, is the active form of thyroid hormone. Although only about 20% of the thyroid hormone produced is T3, it's the form that your cells use to regulate metabolism. T3 influences various bodily functions, including heart rate, digestion, muscle control, brain function, and even bone maintenance.

T3 acts on almost every cell in the body by binding to thyroid hormone receptors within the cells and activating them. This activation leads to an increase in metabolic processes, such as the production of energy, the breakdown of fats, and the regulation of body temperature.

Reverse T3: The Brake Pedal

Reverse T3 (rT3) is a form of T3 that has been altered slightly, rendering it inactive. Think of rT3 as the brake pedal in your metabolic system. It's produced when the body needs to slow down metabolism, such as during times of stress, illness, or caloric restriction. rT3 competes with T3 for binding sites on the thyroid hormone receptors, effectively slowing down the metabolic rate when needed.

While rT3 has a role in helping the body conserve energy during stressful times, an excess of rT3 can lead to symptoms of hypothyroidism, even if TSH, T4 and T3 levels are normal. This condition is often referred to as "thyroid resistance" or "euthyroid sick syndrome."

Factors That Affect Thyroid Function

Often referred to as "the canary in the coal mine", the thyroid is a sensitive gland, and its function can quickly be influenced by various factors, including nutrient deficiencies, stress, toxins, and autoimmune conditions. It is often the first gland that will alert you that something isn't right in your body!

Understanding these factors and watching out for the signs and symptoms, can help you take steps to protect your thyroid and maintain optimal health.

Nutrient Deficiencies

Certain nutrients are essential for thyroid hormone production and conversion. Deficiencies in these nutrients can lead to impaired thyroid function:

- **Iodine:** Iodine is an essential building block of both T3 and T4. Without enough iodine, the thyroid cannot produce sufficient amounts of these hormones. While iodine deficiency is less common in developed countries due to iodized salt, it can still occur in those who avoid salt or consume a diet low in iodine-rich foods like seafood, seaweed, and dairy products.

- **Selenium:** Selenium is crucial for the conversion of T4 into T3. It also helps protect the thyroid from oxidative damage. Low selenium levels can impair this conversion process, leading to low T3 levels and symptoms of hypothyroidism. Conversely, high selenium is toxic.

- **Zinc and Iron:** Both zinc and iron play roles in thyroid hormone synthesis and conversion. Zinc is needed for TSH production, while iron is essential for the enzymes that produce thyroid hormones. Deficiencies in these minerals can contribute to thyroid dysfunction.

- **Vitamin D:** Vitamin D is necessary for the normal functioning of many organs, including the thyroid gland. It is, therefore, not surprising that vitamin D deficiency is considered a risk factor for the development of many thyroid disorders, including autoimmune thyroid diseases and thyroid cancer.

Stress and Cortisol

Chronic stress can have a significant impact on thyroid function. When you're stressed, your body produces cortisol, the stress hormone, which can interfere with thyroid hormone production and conversion. High cortisol levels can suppress TSH, lower the conversion of T4 to T3, and increase the production of rT3, leading to symptoms of hypothyroidism even if thyroid hormone levels appear normal. You will need to address the stress to improve your thyroid health.

Oestrogen

High oestrogen levels can increase the concentration of thyroxine-binding globulin (TBG), a protein that binds to thyroid hormones, resulting in decreased free thyroid hormone levels. This can lead to symptoms of hypothyroidism, such as fatigue, weight gain, and mood swings even if lab results look completely normal.

Toxins and Endocrine Disruptors

Environmental toxins and endocrine disruptors can also negatively affect thyroid function. Chemicals like BPA (found in plastics), pesticides, and heavy metals (like mercury and lead) can interfere with thyroid hormone production and conversion. These toxins can mimic or block thyroid hormones, leading to imbalances and disrupted metabolic processes.

Arsenic is extremely toxic to the whole body including the thyroid. It is found in rice, shellfish and well water. It also used to be used to treat wood, so treated wood should also be considered a source.

Bromine is commonly found in flame-proofing agents, fumigants, some medications, and pool/spa sanitisers. Bromine can displace iodine and affect the synthesis of T4.

Cadmium can also accumulate in the thyroid and affect its function. The most common source is cigarette smoke.

Copper needs to be kept in balance for optimal thyroid function. Copper is known to interfere with the absorption and utilisation of various minerals in the body, including zinc and selenium, which are essential for optimal thyroid function. A deficiency in these minerals can worsen hypothyroidism symptoms and contribute to the overall decline in thyroid health. Too much or too little copper can both impact thyroid function.

Lithium, although an amazing nutrient for the brain, if taken in excess, can concentrate in the thyroid and inhibit thyroidal iodine uptake. It also affects thyroid hormone secretion. The latter effect is critical to the development of hypothyroidism and goitre (noticeable swelling of the thyroid).

Mercury can also bind with cells in the thyroid gland and lead to an under-active thyroid, known as hypothyroidism.

Autoimmune Conditions

Hashimoto's thyroiditis is an autoimmune condition in which the immune system attacks the thyroid gland, leading to chronic inflammation and impaired thyroid function. It's the most common cause of hypothyroidism in developed countries. Many people with Hashimoto's respond well to a gluten free diet and supplements that support the Thyroid. But many people with Hashimoto's will also need medication.

Graves' disease, another autoimmune condition, causes the thyroid to overproduce hormones, leading to hyperthyroidism. Managing autoimmune conditions is crucial for maintaining thyroid health and hormonal balance. People with Graves' disease respond well to a high protein diet with supplemental anti-oxidants along with their medication.

Supporting Thyroid Health

To support your thyroid and maintain optimal hormonal balance, consider the following strategies:

1. **Ensure Adequate Nutrient Intake:** Incorporate iodine-rich foods like seaweed, seafood, and dairy, as well as selenium-rich foods like brazil nuts, eggs, and sunflower seeds, into your diet. Make sure you're getting enough

zinc (from foods like oysters, beef, and pumpkin seeds) and iron (from red meat, lentils, and spinach). Good quality protein is also essential for the amino acid Tyrosine that makes thyroid hormones.

2. **Manage Stress:** Practice stress-reducing techniques like mindfulness, yoga, deep breathing, and regular exercise to help regulate cortisol levels and support thyroid function. You may need to assess your adrenal function to make sure they are not contributing to your thyroid being unwell.

3. **Limit Exposure to Toxins:** Choose organic produce, avoid plastics (especially when heating food), and consider filtering your water to reduce exposure to endocrine disruptors and heavy metals.

4. **Monitor Thyroid Function:** Regular check-ups with your healthcare provider can help monitor thyroid function and ensure that any imbalances are addressed early.

Symptoms of a thyroid imbalance:

Thyroid hormone imbalances can manifest in various ways depending on whether the thyroid is overactive (hyperthyroidism) or underactive (hypothyroidism). Here's a breakdown of the main symptoms for each condition:

Hypothyroidism (Underactive Thyroid)

Hypothyroidism occurs when the thyroid gland doesn't produce enough thyroid hormones. This slows down the body's metabolism and can lead to a variety of symptoms:

1. **Fatigue:** Persistent tiredness and lack of energy, even after a full night's sleep.

2. **Weight Gain:** Unexplained weight gain or difficulty losing weight, despite a healthy diet and exercise.

3. **Cold Intolerance:** Feeling unusually cold or having a lower body temperature, even in warm environments.

4. **Dry Skin and Hair:** Skin may become dry, rough, and flaky, and hair can become brittle, dry, and prone to falling out.

5. **Constipation:** Slowed digestion leading to constipation or infrequent bowel movements.

6. **Depression:** Feeling sad, depressed, or having a low mood, often accompanied by a lack of interest in activities.

7. **Memory Problems:** Difficulty concentrating, forgetfulness, or brain fog.

8. **Muscle Weakness and Joint Pain:** General muscle weakness, aches, stiffness, or joint pain.

9. **Slow Heart Rate:** A slower-than-normal heart rate (bradycardia).

10. **Heavy or Irregular Periods:** In women, menstrual cycles may become heavier, longer, or irregular.

11. **Hoarseness:** A hoarse voice or a feeling of a lump in the throat.

12. **Swelling:** Puffiness in the face, particularly around the eyes, and swelling in the hands and feet.

13. **Loss of eyebrow hairs:** A common sign that the thyroid is not balanced is the loss of hair from the outside part of your eyebrows.

Hyperthyroidism (Overactive Thyroid)

Hyperthyroidism occurs when the thyroid gland produces too much thyroid hormone, speeding up the body's metabolism and leading to these symptoms:

1. **Weight Loss:** Unintentional weight loss despite having a normal or increased appetite.

2. **Rapid or Irregular Heartbeat:** A fast heart rate (tachycardia), palpitations, or irregular heartbeats.

3. **Nervousness and Anxiety:** Feeling unusually anxious, jittery, or nervous, often with restlessness.

4. **Irritability:** Increased irritability or mood swings.

5. **Heat Intolerance:** Feeling overly warm or sweaty, even in cool environments.

6. **Tremors:** Shaking or trembling hands and fingers.

7. **Increased Appetite:** A higher-than-normal appetite, sometimes accompanied by weight loss.

8. **Frequent Bowel Movements:** More frequent or loose bowel movements, sometimes leading to diarrhoea.

9. **Sleep Problems:** Difficulty falling asleep, staying asleep, or having restless sleep (insomnia).

10. **Muscle Weakness:** Weakness in muscles, particularly in the thighs and upper arms.

11. **Menstrual Changes:** In women, menstrual periods may become lighter, shorter, or less frequent.

12. **Bulging Eyes (Exophthalmos):** In cases of Graves' disease, a form of hyperthyroidism, the eyes may appear enlarged or bulging.

13. **Thinning Skin and Hair:** Skin can become thin and fragile, and hair may thin or fall out.

Testing:

Thyroid hormones are best tested using blood. You can do basic thyroid function, or if you suspect auto immunity or stress as an issue, you should also assess the antibodies and Reverse T3 and overall adrenal function.

You can also use a test that assesses the toxic and essential nutrients that can affect thyroid health.

In functional medicine, the focus is on identifying and addressing the root causes of health issues and optimising overall well-being. When it comes to thyroid hormones, functional medicine practitioners often use narrower, more optimised reference ranges compared to conventional labs. This is because they aim to catch and address imbalances before they develop into more significant health problems. Before testing your thyroid hormones, please stop using supplements that contain Biotin, as this has been shown to affect thyroid test results.

Here's a comparison between the conventional lab reference ranges and the optimal ranges commonly used in functional medicine:

1. Thyroid-Stimulating Hormone (TSH)

- **Best tested first thing in the morning**
- **Conventional Lab Range:** Typically 0.5 to 4.5 mIU/L (or sometimes up to 5.0 mIU/L) but these ranges can vary from lab to lab. Ideally, use the same lab for re testing.
- **Functional Medicine Optimal Range:** 1.0 to 2.5 mIU/L

○ **Perspective:** TSH is often considered the primary screening tool for thyroid function. Functional medicine practitioners prefer to see TSH in the 1.0 to 2.5 mIU/L range because levels outside this range, even if still "normal" by conventional standards, might indicate a suboptimal thyroid function.

2. Free T4 (Thyroxine)

- **Conventional Lab Range:** Approximately 0.8 to 1.8 ng/dL
- **Functional Medicine Optimal Range:** 1.0 to 1.5 ng/dL

  - **Perspective:** Free T4 represents the amount of unbound, active thyroid hormone in the blood. Functional medicine aims to keep free T4 in a mid-to-upper range, suggesting that the thyroid is adequately producing hormones without over or underproduction.

3. Free T3 (Triiodothyronine)

- **Conventional Lab Range:** Approximately 2.3 to 4.2 pg/mL
- **Functional Medicine Optimal Range:** 3.2 to 4.2 pg/mL

  - **Perspective:** Free T3 is the active form of thyroid hormone that exerts the most significant effects at the cellular level. Functional medicine practitioners often prioritize free T3 levels, as they can be a better indicator of how well the thyroid is functioning and how well T4 is converting to T3.

4. Reverse T3 (rT3)

- **Conventional Lab Range:** Approximately 10 to 24 ng/dL
- **Functional Medicine Optimal Range:** 10 to 15 ng/dL, or a ratio of free T3 to reverse T3 above 20
  - **Perspective:** Reverse T3 is an inactive form of T3 that can block the action of active T3 by binding to T3 receptors. High levels of rT3 can indicate issues like chronic stress, inflammation, or nutrient deficiencies. Functional medicine practitioners often assess the free T3/reverse T3 ratio to evaluate thyroid function comprehensively.

5. Thyroid Antibodies

- **Thyroid Peroxidase Antibodies (TPOAb)**
- **Thyroglobulin Antibodies (TgAb)**
- **Conventional Lab Range:**
  - TPOAb: <35 IU/mL
  - TgAb: <20 IU/mL
- **Functional Medicine Optimal Range:** As close to zero as possible

○ **Perspective:** Even slightly elevated thyroid antibodies can indicate autoimmune thyroid disease, such as Hashimoto's thyroiditis or Graves' disease. Functional medicine practitioners aim to reduce these antibodies as much as possible through lifestyle, diet, and targeted interventions to prevent or manage autoimmune thyroid conditions.

Key Points in the Functional Medicine Approach:

- **Context Matters:** Functional medicine practitioners consider the patient's symptoms and health history, not just lab results. A person might have "normal" thyroid lab results but still experience symptoms of thyroid dysfunction, prompting further investigation.

- **Nutrient Optimisation:** Nutrients like iodine, selenium, zinc, and vitamin D are critical for thyroid function. Functional medicine often includes assessing and optimising these nutrients. Natural desiccated thyroid can be prescribed by a qualified professional and will need consistent monitoring.

- **Comprehensive Testing:** Beyond TSH, a full thyroid panel including Free T4, Free T3, Reverse T3, and thyroid antibodies is often recommended to get a complete picture of thyroid health. Including the nutrients and metals that can impact thyroid health is a useful add on to a thyroid test, as well as assessing adrenal health.

Conclusion:

The optimal ranges used in functional medicine are often narrower and more targeted than conventional lab ranges. This approach aims to detect and address thyroid imbalances early, potentially preventing more significant thyroid dysfunction and improving overall health. If you suspect thyroid issues but your labs fall within the "normal" range, it may be beneficial to consult with a functional medicine practitioner who can help you explore these optimal ranges and additional testing.

Your thyroid gland is a key player in your body's metabolic symphony and understanding how its hormones work and what influences them, is essential for maintaining overall health. By supporting your thyroid with proper nutrition, stress management, and a toxin-free environment, you can help ensure that your body's metabolism stays in harmony, allowing you to feel energetic, vibrant, and healthy.

Chapter 5

The Adrenals: Navigating the Stress Hormones

Stress can make any instrument in your orchestra go out of tune! In our fast-paced world, stress has become a common part of everyday life. While some stress is normal and even beneficial, chronic stress can have a profound impact on your health, particularly on your adrenal glands and the hormones they produce. The adrenal glands, perched atop your kidneys, are responsible for producing hormones that help you cope with stress, regulate your metabolism, and maintain energy levels. In this chapter, we'll explore the adrenal hormones, how they respond to stress, and what you can do to support your adrenal health. If there is anything that can make your orchestra sound more like a cacophony than a melody, stress would be it!

Your nervous system has 2 states, the first, is the "rest and digest, feed and breed" *Parasympathetic state*, where rest, digestion and reproduction are a priority. Then there is the second, the "fright, fight or flight" *Sympathetic state*, where your body prioritises running away or fighting its way out of a dangerous situation. Digestion and reproduction are no longer the priority. Unfortunately, your body can't tell the difference between being attacked by a tiger and work stress or financial stress or relationship stress, the response will be the same. This is why relaxation techniques come up often as a way to reset your nervous system and your adrenal hormones, which will then affect your other hormones and digestion.

Although we will focus on the adrenal hormones, stress itself can also impact the health of the stomach, by making the stomach less acidic, which has a knock-on effect on the rest of the gut, especially if you aren't eating mindfully or chewing well at the same time. Stress also makes the body remove vital electrolytes, which is why people often crave salt when they are chronically stressed. Sometimes replacing the electrolytes (there are many good, sugar free, balance formulas on the market) can help with some of the symptoms.

The Adrenal Hormones: Cortisol, Adrenaline, and More

Whether the stress you are experiencing is coming from outside of yourself, such as a natural disaster or work deadline, or whether it is coming from within, like the anxiety experienced from public speaking or just ruminating on past mistakes, it is the adrenal glands that help us to adapt and survive. The adrenals are also key regulators of blood sugar, insulin, digestion and inflammation, and play a major role in mood and mental focus, stamina and sleep cycles.

The adrenal glands produce several key hormones that play vital roles in your body's response to stress, energy production, and overall well-being. Let's take a closer look at the most important adrenal hormones and their functions.

Adrenaline and Noradrenaline: The Rapid Responders

Adrenaline (also known as epinephrine) and noradrenaline (norepinephrine) are hormones produced by the adrenal medulla, the inner part of the adrenal glands. These hormones are released in response to acute stress and are responsible for the "fight-or-flight" response.

Adrenaline increases heart rate, elevates blood pressure, and boosts energy supplies, preparing your body to either face the threat or flee from it. Noradrenaline works alongside adrenaline, helping to maintain blood pressure and increase blood flow to essential organs. While these hormones are crucial for survival, chronic activation can lead to symptoms like anxiety, high blood pressure, and heart palpitations.

DHEA (Dehydroepiandrosterone)
A precursor and balancer of hormones

DHEA is a vital adrenal hormone that helps produce sex hormones, balance stress, and support overall health. It declines with age, and maintaining optimal DHEA levels is essential for energy, immunity, and mood balance. Its interplay with cortisol is key in managing the body's response to stress, providing a counterbalance to the potentially harmful effects of chronic stress and aging.

1. Role and Function of DHEA

- **Precursor to Other Hormones:** DHEA is often referred to as a "prohormone" because the body converts it into androgens (like testosterone) and oestrogens (like estradiol), the primary male and female sex hormones, respectively. It's one of the main sources of sex hormone production in both men and women, especially after middle age when the production of sex hormones declines.

- **Stress Response and Adrenal Function:** Produced by the adrenal cortex, DHEA is a part of the body's response to stress, along with other hormones like cortisol. However, while cortisol is typically known as the "stress hormone," DHEA has a more balancing effect—helping to mitigate some of the negative effects of chronic stress and high cortisol levels. DHEA helps to support the body's immune system, mood, and overall energy levels.

2. DHEA Levels Over Time

- **Peak and Decline:** DHEA levels peak in early adulthood, around the age of 20 to 25, and gradually decline as you age. By the time most people reach their 70s or 80s, DHEA levels can be as much as 80–90% lower than in youth.

- This decline is part of the natural aging process and can contribute to age-related changes like decreased bone density, reduced muscle mass, and lower libido.

3. DHEA and Stress

- **Balancing Cortisol:** DHEA acts in balance with cortisol, the primary stress hormone. While cortisol helps the body deal with acute stress, prolonged high cortisol levels can lead to negative effects such as immune suppression, weight gain, and mood disturbances. DHEA can counter some of these effects by reducing inflammation, improving immune function, and enhancing well-being.

- **Chronic Stress:** In cases of chronic stress, the adrenal glands can become overworked, leading to lower levels of DHEA and elevated cortisol. This imbalance can contribute to feelings of fatigue, poor immune response, and emotional instability.

4. Benefits of DHEA

- **Energy and Vitality:** Adequate DHEA levels are associated with higher energy, improved mood, and better mental clarity.

- **Bone Health:** DHEA contributes to maintaining bone density, which is especially important in older adults at risk of osteoporosis.

- **Immune Function:** DHEA helps support the immune system, making it important for overall health and resistance to infections.

- **Sexual Health:** Since DHEA is a precursor to sex hormones, it plays a role in maintaining libido and reproductive health, particularly as people age.

5. DHEA Supplementation

- Due to its role in aging and stress management, some individuals take DHEA supplements to try to boost hormone levels. However, DHEA supplementation should be done cautiously and under medical supervision, as imbalances can lead to side effects like acne, hair loss, or changes in mood.

Cortisol: The Long Term Stress Hormone

Cortisol is perhaps the most well-known adrenal hormone, often referred to as the "stress hormone." Produced by the adrenal cortex, cortisol helps your body respond to stressful situations by increasing blood sugar levels, suppressing the immune system, and aiding in metabolism.

In the short term, cortisol is beneficial—it helps you react quickly in a fight-or-flight situation. However, when stress becomes chronic, cortisol levels can remain elevated, leading to a range of health issues. Chronic high cortisol levels can contribute to weight gain (particularly around the abdomen), high blood pressure, anxiety, sleep disturbances, and weakened immune function.

Cortisone, Free Cortisol and Metabolised Cortisol

Measured in a dried urine test, **cortisone**, **free cortisol**, and **metabolised cortisol** represent different forms and functions of cortisol, a key hormone in the body's stress response. Here's a breakdown of each term and their significance:

1. Cortisone

- **What it is**: Cortisone is an inactive form of cortisol. The body can convert cortisol (the active form) into cortisone to regulate cortisol levels and reduce its biological effects. What this means, is that your body can choose in any instant to change the amount of active cortisol available from the adrenals glands. So if your adrenal glands have been pumping loads of cortisol into your body, but your body only really needs a small amount, it can de activate some to cortisone.

- **Measurement**: Measuring cortisone in urine provides insights into how much of the active cortisol has been produced and then converted into its inactive form. High or low cortisone levels can indicate how efficiently your body is managing stress or inflammatory responses.

- **Significance**: This shows how your body might be trying to reduce the effects of cortisol by converting it to cortisone, offering clues about overall cortisol regulation and potential adrenal function.

2. Free Cortisol

- **What it is**: Free cortisol refers to the small portion of cortisol that is not bound to proteins in the blood, and is biologically active. This is the fraction of cortisol that is available to interact with receptors and enact effects like regulating metabolism, immune response, and stress reactions. Most cortisol is bound to a protein util it is needed and made "free".

- **Measurement**: Free cortisol levels measured in saliva or urine reflect the active cortisol circulating in your system at the time of collection. It provides a snapshot of how much cortisol is immediately available to affect the body.

- **Significance**: Free cortisol is critical for assessing adrenal function and the immediate cortisol activity. High levels could indicate stress, while low levels could suggest adrenal fatigue or low cortisol production.

3. Metabolised Cortisol (Total Cortisol Metabolites)

- **What it is**: Metabolised cortisol is the sum of all cortisol that has been broken down by the liver and processed for excretion. It represents the total cortisol output over time, rather than just the free or active cortisol circulating in the system.

- **Measurement**: This measurement shows the total cortisol that has been produced and processed by the body, including both free cortisol and bound cortisol that has been metabolised and rendered inactive.

- **Significance**: Metabolised cortisol helps to understand overall cortisol production. If free cortisol is low but metabolised cortisol is high, it may suggest that the body is making plenty of cortisol but clearing it out quickly. Conversely, low metabolised cortisol with low free cortisol can point to low overall cortisol production.

Key Differences:

- **Cortisol:** The biologically active stress hormone.

- **Free Cortisol** is the active form that is immediately usable by the body, indicating current stress or adrenal function.

- **Metabolised Cortisol** reflects the total amount of cortisol that has been produced and processed, providing a picture of overall cortisol production and turnover.

- **Cortisone** is the inactive form of cortisol, giving insight into how the body is deactivating cortisol.

These values together give a more comprehensive understanding of how the body is managing stress, adrenal health, and overall hormonal balance.

The Diurnal Dance between Melatonin and Cortisol

Although melatonin is not a stress hormone made by the adrenal glands, let's look at the relationship that Cortisol has with Melatonin as these 2 hormones dance closely together throughout a daily cycle.

Cortisol and melatonin are two key hormones that help regulate your sleep-wake cycle, working in opposition to each other to maintain balance. Here's how their levels ebb and flow throughout the day, from waking to sleep:

1. Morning: High Cortisol, Low Melatonin

- **Cortisol** peaks early in the morning, typically around **6 to 8 a.m.**, to help you wake up and start your day. This rise in cortisol is part of the **"Cortisol Awakening Response"** (CAR). It helps you feel more alert, increases energy, and gets your body ready to deal with the demands of the day by boosting blood sugar and metabolism. Measuring the CAR is a good way to assess just how healthy your adrenals are. This is done using saliva samples done on waking, 30 minutes after waking and then 30 minutes after that. Any deviation from the normal up and down curve can indicate that your adrenals need help.

- During this time, **melatonin** is at its lowest levels. Melatonin, which is the body's "sleep hormone," decreases sharply in the early morning to allow for wakefulness.

2. Daytime: Moderate Cortisol, Low Melatonin

- Throughout the day, cortisol remains at a **moderate level** but gradually decreases. This hormone helps manage stress, keeps energy steady, and supports various body functions, but it is no longer at its morning peak.

- **Melatonin** stays low during daylight hours. Exposure to sunlight suppresses melatonin production, which helps you stay awake and alert.

3. Late Afternoon to Early Evening: Declining Cortisol

- In the **late afternoon and early evening**, cortisol continues to decline as your body prepares to wind down. Energy levels naturally dip, and this is why you may feel a little sluggish during these hours.

- **Melatonin** remains low but will start to rise soon as the light fades.

4. Evening: Rising Melatonin, Lower Cortisol

- As night approaches and it gets darker, **melatonin levels begin to rise**, typically around **8 to 10 p.m.**. This increase signals to your body that it's time to prepare for sleep.

- **Cortisol** reaches its lowest levels in the evening. With low cortisol and rising melatonin, your body starts to relax, your metabolism slows down, and you begin to feel sleepy.

5. Night: High Melatonin, Low Cortisol

- **Melatonin** peaks during the night, usually between **midnight and 2 a.m.**, which helps maintain a deep, restorative sleep. It keeps your body's internal clock in sync and promotes a restful night. But be warned, light, especially blue light (from your phone) can switch off the supply of melatonin!

- **Cortisol** stays very low while you sleep, allowing your body to rest and recover. However, it starts to rise again toward morning in preparation for waking.

6. Pre-Dawn: Melatonin Drops, Cortisol Rises

- In the early morning hours, around **3 to 6 a.m.**, **melatonin levels begin to drop** as light exposure increases (even if it's just subtle sunrise light). This helps your body start to transition toward wakefulness.

- At the same time, **cortisol** begins to rise again, gearing up for the new day and ensuring you feel alert when you wake up.

Summary of that night and day dance:

- **Cortisol** is high in the morning to wake you up, decreases throughout the day, and is at its lowest at night.

- **Melatonin** is low during the day, starts rising in the evening, peaks at night to promote sleep, and then decreases again before morning.

This natural ebb and flow of cortisol and melatonin is crucial for maintaining a healthy sleep-wake cycle, keeping you energized during the day and restful at night.

How Stress Affects the Adrenal Glands

Your body is equipped to handle short-term stress, but when stress becomes chronic, it can take a toll on your adrenal glands and the hormones they produce. Here's how chronic stress affects your adrenal function:

Adrenal Fatigue: When the Adrenals Can't Keep Up

Adrenal fatigue is a term often used to describe a condition in which the adrenal glands become overworked due to chronic stress, leading to a decline in cortisol production. While "adrenal fatigue" is not a recognised medical diagnosis, the symptoms are real and often overlap with other conditions such as hypothyroidism, chronic fatigue syndrome, and depression.

Symptoms of adrenal fatigue can include fatigue, difficulty waking up in the morning, cravings for salty or sweet foods, reliance on caffeine for energy, and a weakened immune system. The idea behind adrenal fatigue is that chronic stress exhausts the adrenal glands, making them less capable of producing adequate levels of cortisol and other hormones.

The HPA Axis: The Stress Response System

The hypothalamic-pituitary-adrenal (HPA) axis is the body's central stress response system. When you encounter a stressful situation, the hypothalamus in your brain signals the pituitary gland to release adrenocorticotropic hormone (ACTH). ACTH then prompts the adrenal glands to produce cortisol.

Chronic stress can dysregulate the HPA axis, leading to either excessive cortisol production or insufficient cortisol production over time. Dysregulation of the HPA axis is associated with a variety of health issues, including anxiety, depression, insomnia, and metabolic disorders.

Supporting Your Adrenal Health

Given the critical role that adrenal hormones play in managing stress and maintaining energy levels, it's important to support your adrenal glands through lifestyle choices and stress management techniques.

Nutrition for Adrenal Support

A balanced diet rich in whole foods can provide the nutrients your adrenal glands need to function properly:

- **B Vitamins:** B vitamins, particularly B5 (pantothenic acid) and B6 (pyridoxil-5-phosphate), are essential for adrenal hormone production. Foods like eggs, poultry, fish, whole grains, and legumes are excellent sources of B vitamins.

- **Vitamin C:** The adrenal glands contain one of the highest concentrations of vitamin C in the body, which is used to produce cortisol. Foods rich in vitamin C include citrus fruits, berries, bell peppers, and broccoli.

- **Magnesium:** Magnesium helps regulate the body's stress response and can support adrenal health. Include magnesium-rich foods like dark leafy greens, nuts, seeds, and whole grains in your diet.

- **Healthy Fats:** Adrenal hormones are steroid hormones, which means they're made from cholesterol. Healthy fats, such as those found in avocados, nuts, seeds, and olive oil, provide the raw materials for hormone production.

Stress Management Techniques

Managing stress is crucial for maintaining healthy adrenal function. Consider incorporating the following practices into your routine:

- **Mindfulness and Meditation:** These practices can help reduce stress and lower cortisol levels. Even just a few minutes a day can make a difference.

- **Regular Exercise:** Moderate exercise, such as walking, yoga, or swimming, can help reduce stress and improve overall adrenal function. However, be mindful not to over-exercise, as excessive physical stress can further strain the adrenals.

- **Sleep:** Adequate sleep is essential for adrenal recovery. Aim for 7-9 hours of quality sleep per night and establish a regular sleep routine.

- **Social Support:** Spending time with loved ones and fostering strong social connections can help buffer the effects of stress and support adrenal health.

- **Limiting Stimulants**: Caffeine and sugar can exacerbate stress and overwork the adrenal glands. While it's okay to enjoy these in moderation, relying on them for energy can create a vicious cycle of stress and adrenal strain. Consider reducing your intake and replacing caffeinated beverages with herbal teas or water and choose whole fruits over sugary snacks.

Symptoms:

Adrenal hormone imbalances can manifest in various ways depending on whether the adrenal glands are overactive or underactive. These imbalances often involve cortisol and DHEA, two critical adrenal hormones that play significant roles in stress response, metabolism, immune function, and overall well-being.

Overactive Adrenal Glands (Excess Cortisol)

When the adrenal glands produce too much cortisol, it can lead to a condition known as **Cushing's syndrome** or other stress-related disorders. Symptoms of excess cortisol include:

1. **Weight Gain:** Particularly in the abdomen, face ("moon face"), and upper back ("buffalo hump").

2. **High Blood Pressure:** Cortisol can raise blood pressure, leading to hypertension.

3. **Mood Changes:** Increased anxiety, irritability, and depression are common.

4. **Sleep Disturbances:** Difficulty falling asleep or staying asleep, insomnia.

5. **Fatigue:** Despite high cortisol, there can be feelings of exhaustion, particularly in the afternoon.

6. **Muscle Weakness:** Weakness, especially in the legs.

7. **Increased Blood Sugar Levels:** Cortisol raises blood glucose levels, increasing the risk of insulin resistance or diabetes.

8. **Weakened Immune System:** Frequent infections or longer recovery times.

9. **Osteoporosis:** Loss of bone density over time.

10. **Thinning Skin and Easy Bruising:** Skin becomes more fragile and slower to heal.

Underactive Adrenal Glands (Low Cortisol)

Low cortisol production, as seen in **Adrenal Insufficiency** or **Addison's Disease**, can lead to the following symptoms:

1. **Chronic Fatigue:** Extreme tiredness that doesn't improve with rest.

2. **Weight Loss:** Unintentional weight loss, often accompanied by decreased appetite.

3. **Low Blood Pressure:** Dizziness or fainting due to hypotension.

4. **Salt Cravings:** A strong desire for salty foods due to low sodium levels.

5. **Low Blood Sugar:** Hypoglycaemia, causing shakiness, irritability, and light-headedness.

6. **Muscle Weakness:** Persistent muscle fatigue and weakness.

7. **Darkening of the Skin:** Hyperpigmentation, especially in areas exposed to friction (such as elbows, knees, and knuckles).

8. **Mood Changes:** Depression, irritability, and apathy.

9. **Digestive Issues:** Nausea, vomiting, diarrhoea, and abdominal pain.

10. **Joint and Muscle Pain:** Generalised aches and pains.

Assessing Adrenal Hormones: Cortisol and DHEA

1. Cortisol Testing: Free vs. Metabolised Cortisol

Cortisol can be measured in several forms, with free and metabolized cortisol providing different insights:

- **Free Cortisol:**
  - **Saliva:** Measures the free, active cortisol at specific times during the day (usually four samples—morning, noon, afternoon, and night) to assess the diurnal rhythm. It's useful for identifying how cortisol levels fluctuate throughout the day.
  - **Dried Urine Test:** Measures free cortisol in urine at 4 points in the day, providing a comprehensive look at daily cortisol production and its pattern. Dried urine would also include cortisone and metabolised cortisol.

- **Metabolised Cortisol:**
  - **Dried Urine Test:** Measures the total amount of cortisol that has been metabolised by the liver and excreted in the urine. It gives an overall picture of

adrenal output and how well the body processes cortisol. Assessing this with salivary free cortisol gives a more accurate idea of how the adrenals are coping.

Factors Influencing Cortisol Results:

- **Stress Levels:** Acute or chronic stress or injuries can significantly affect cortisol levels.

- **Sleep Patterns:** Poor sleep or irregular sleep-wake cycles can disrupt cortisol production.

- **Diet:** Caffeine, sugar, and alcohol can influence cortisol levels.

- **Exercise:** Intense physical activity, especially late in the day, can alter cortisol levels.

- **Medications:** Steroids and other medications can affect cortisol production and metabolism.

2. DHEA vs. DHEA-S Testing

- **DHEA (Dehydroepiandrosterone):** This is the active form of the hormone. It is best assessed through blood, saliva, or urine tests, usually in the morning.

- **DHEA-S (Dehydroepiandrosterone Sulphate):** This is the sulphated, more stable, and longer-lasting form of DHEA, typically measured in blood tests to provide a more accurate reflection of adrenal activity over time.

Factors Influencing DHEA Results:

- **Age:** DHEA levels peak in early adulthood and decline with age.

- **Gender:** Levels are generally higher in men than women.

- **Stress:** Chronic stress can deplete DHEA levels.

- **Nutrition:** Nutrient deficiencies (e.g., zinc, vitamin C) can impact DHEA production.

- **Exercise:** Regular moderate exercise can support healthy DHEA levels.

Factors Influencing DHEA-s Results:

- **Low cysteine:** Poor liver function or a deficiency in Cysteine can affect the conversion of DHEA to DHEA-s

- **Inflammation**

- **Lipopolysaccharides (LPS)**

- **Liquorice root**

- **Progestin**

Adaptogens Help the Adrenals to Adapt to stress better

Adaptogens are a unique group of herbs and natural substances that help the body adapt to stress, support adrenal health, and promote overall balance and resilience. They are particularly valuable for maintaining and restoring adrenal function, especially in individuals experiencing chronic stress, burnout, or adrenal fatigue.

How Adaptogens Work

Adaptogens exert a balancing effect on the body, particularly on the hypothalamic-pituitary-adrenal (HPA) axis, which regulates the body's stress response. They do this by modulating the release of stress hormones like cortisol and helping the body maintain homeostasis during stressful situations. Unlike stimulants, which can overtax the adrenal glands, adaptogens provide a non-specific resistance to stress, improving the body's ability to cope without depleting energy reserves.

Key Adaptogens for Adrenal Health

1. Ashwagandha (Withania somnifera)

- **Role in Adrenal Health:** Ashwagandha is one of the most well-known adaptogens for supporting adrenal function. It helps regulate cortisol levels, reducing high cortisol in times of chronic stress and improving overall resilience. It also supports thyroid function, which is closely linked to adrenal health.

- **Benefits:** Reduces anxiety, improves sleep quality, enhances energy levels, and supports immune function.

- **Mechanism:** Ashwagandha modulates the HPA axis, balancing cortisol production and promoting a calm, stable mood.

2. Rhodiola Rosea

- **Role in Adrenal Health:** Rhodiola is known for its ability to enhance mental and physical performance under stress. It helps prevent adrenal exhaustion by improving the body's stress response, particularly in high-pressure situations.

- **Benefits:** Increases stamina, reduces fatigue, boosts mood, and supports cognitive function.

- **Mechanism:** Rhodiola influences the release of stress hormones while protecting the brain and heart from the harmful effects of stress.

3. Holy Basil (Tulsi)

- **Role in Adrenal Health:** Holy Basil is revered in Ayurvedic medicine for its calming effects on the mind and body. It helps to reduce stress and anxiety while supporting adrenal balance.

- **Benefits:** Reduces stress-related symptoms, improves mood, and supports healthy blood sugar levels.

- **Mechanism:** Holy Basil modulates cortisol levels and helps balance neurotransmitters, contributing to overall stress resilience.

4. Panax Ginseng (Asian Ginseng)

- **Role in Adrenal Health:** Panax Ginseng is a powerful adaptogen known for its stimulating effects, which can help restore energy and vitality in cases of adrenal fatigue. It's particularly effective in boosting physical performance and reducing stress.

- **Benefits:** Enhances energy, improves mental clarity, and supports immune function.

- **Mechanism:** Panax Ginseng supports the HPA axis, improves circulation, and balances cortisol levels, particularly in individuals with low energy due to adrenal insufficiency.

5. Eleuthero (Siberian Ginseng)

- **Role in Adrenal Health:** Eleuthero is an adaptogen that enhances the body's resilience to stress and supports adrenal recovery. It is particularly useful for improving stamina and endurance.

- **Benefits:** Increases energy, supports cognitive function, and enhances physical performance.

- **Mechanism:** Eleuthero helps regulate the stress response by supporting adrenal function and stabilizing cortisol levels.

6. liquorice Root (Glycyrrhiza glabra)

- **Role in Adrenal Health:** liquorice root is unique among adaptogens because it specifically supports adrenal function by prolonging the half-life of cortisol, making it beneficial for individuals with low cortisol levels.

- **Benefits:** Supports energy levels, reduces fatigue, and enhances stress resilience.

- **Mechanism:** liquorice root inhibits the enzyme 11β-hydroxysteroid dehydrogenase type 2, which breaks down cortisol, thereby extending its action in the body. This can be particularly helpful for individuals with low cortisol but should be used cautiously in those with high blood pressure or high cortisol levels.

Benefits of Adaptogens for Adrenal Health

1. **Balancing Cortisol Levels:** Adaptogens help to regulate cortisol production, whether it's too high or too low. By modulating the body's stress response, they help maintain optimal cortisol levels throughout the day.

2. **Supporting Energy Levels:** Chronic stress and adrenal fatigue often lead to depleted energy. Adaptogens can

help restore vitality by improving the efficiency of energy production and reducing the overall stress burden on the body.

3. **Enhancing Mental and Physical Performance:** Many adaptogens improve cognitive function, focus, and physical stamina, which are often compromised when adrenal health is poor.

4. **Improving Sleep and Reducing Anxiety:** By calming the nervous system and balancing stress hormones, adaptogens can improve sleep quality and reduce anxiety, which are crucial for adrenal recovery.

5. **Protecting Against the Effects of Chronic Stress:** Adaptogens have antioxidant and anti-inflammatory properties that help protect the body from the damaging effects of chronic stress, including oxidative stress and inflammation, which can further tax the adrenal glands.

Conclusion:

Adrenal hormone imbalances, whether due to overactive or underactive adrenal glands, can cause a wide range of symptoms that affect overall health and quality of life. Testing both free and metabolised cortisol, as well as DHEA and DHEA-S levels, provides a comprehensive view of adrenal function.

Functional medicine practitioners often use narrower, more optimal ranges to detect and address imbalances before they develop into more significant health issues. Understanding the factors that influence these results can help tailor interventions to restore adrenal health and hormonal balance.

Adaptogens are powerful tools for supporting adrenal health, particularly in times of chronic stress or adrenal fatigue. They work by balancing the body's stress response, supporting cortisol production, and enhancing overall resilience. Each adaptogen has its unique properties and mechanisms, making it important to choose the right one based on individual needs and symptoms. When used properly, adaptogens can significantly contribute to restoring adrenal function, improving energy levels, and enhancing overall well-being.

Your adrenal glands play a vital role in helping you navigate life's stressors. By understanding how they function and what impacts them, you can take proactive steps to support your adrenal health. Managing stress, eating a balanced diet, and incorporating healthy lifestyle practices can go a long way in maintaining your energy levels, supporting your immune system, and promoting overall well-being.

Chapter 6

Glucose Metabolism: The Rhythm of Blood Sugar and the effect on Hormones

Glucose regulation, also known as sugar metabolism, is a fundamental process that provides your body with the energy it needs to function. At the centre of this process is the delicate balance between the hormones insulin and glucagon, which work together to regulate your blood sugar levels. In this chapter, we'll explore how glucose metabolism works, the role of these key hormones, and how lifestyle choices can impact your blood sugar balance.

The Basics of Glucose Metabolism

Glucose is a type of sugar that comes from the carbohydrates you eat. It's one of the primary sources of energy for your cells, especially for your brain, muscles, and other tissues. When you eat carbohydrates, your digestive system breaks them down into glucose, which then enters your bloodstream. The challenge for your body is to keep blood glucose levels within a narrow range, ensuring that your cells have enough energy without allowing blood sugar levels to get too high or too low.

The Role of Insulin

Insulin is a hormone produced by the pancreas in response to rising blood glucose levels. Think of insulin as a key that unlocks the doors of your cells, allowing glucose to enter and be used for energy.

Here's how insulin works:

1. **After a Meal:** When you eat a meal, particularly one high in carbohydrates, your blood glucose levels rise. In response, the pancreas releases insulin into the bloodstream.

2. **Glucose Uptake:** Insulin binds to receptors on the surface of cells, signalling them to take in glucose from the bloodstream. This process lowers blood glucose levels and provides cells with the energy they need.

3. **Storage:** Insulin also promotes the storage of excess glucose in the liver and muscles in the form of glycogen, a storage form of glucose. If there's still extra glucose after glycogen stores are full, insulin helps convert it into fat for long-term energy storage.

The Role of Glucagon

While insulin helps lower blood sugar levels, glucagon has the opposite effect. Glucagon is another hormone produced by the pancreas, and its main job is to raise blood glucose levels when they drop too low.

Here's how glucagon works:

1. **Between Meals:** When you haven't eaten for a while and your blood glucose levels start to decline, the pancreas releases glucagon into the bloodstream.

2. **Glycogen Breakdown:** Glucagon signals the liver to break down glycogen into glucose, which is then released into the bloodstream to raise blood glucose levels and provide energy.

3. **Gluconeogenesis:** If glycogen stores are depleted, glucagon also stimulates a process called gluconeogenesis, where the liver produces glucose from non-carbohydrate sources, such as amino acids.

Together, insulin and glucagon maintain a balance, ensuring that your blood sugar levels stay within a healthy range.

Factors That Impact Glucose Metabolism

Several factors can influence how well your body manages glucose metabolism, including diet, physical activity, sleep, and stress.

Diet and Blood Sugar

What you eat has a direct impact on your blood sugar levels. Different types of foods affect glucose metabolism in different ways:

- **Simple Carbohydrates:** Foods high in simple carbohydrates, such as sugary snacks, white bread, and soda, cause a rapid spike in blood glucose levels, leading to a quick release of insulin. This can result in a sharp drop in blood sugar (a "sugar crash") shortly after, leaving you feeling tired and hungry again.

- **Complex Carbohydrates:** Foods high in complex carbohydrates, such as whole grains, legumes, and vegetables, break down more slowly, leading to a gradual rise in blood glucose levels. This slower digestion helps maintain steady blood sugar levels and provides a more sustained source of energy.

- **Proteins and Fats:** Including proteins and healthy fats in your meals can slow down the digestion of carbohydrates, leading to a more gradual release of glucose into the bloodstream. This helps prevent sharp spikes and crashes in blood sugar levels.

Physical Activity

Exercise plays a crucial role in glucose metabolism. When you exercise, your muscles use glucose for energy, which helps lower blood sugar levels. Regular physical activity also improves insulin sensitivity, meaning your cells become more responsive to insulin, allowing glucose to be used more efficiently.

Different types of exercise have varying effects on glucose metabolism:

- **Aerobic Exercise:** Activities like walking, jogging, swimming, and cycling help lower blood glucose levels both during and after exercise.

- **Resistance Training:** Weightlifting and other forms of strength training can increase muscle mass, which enhances your body's ability to store glucose and improves insulin sensitivity.

- **High-Intensity Interval Training (HIIT):** HIIT involves short bursts of intense exercise followed by periods of rest. This type of exercise can significantly improve insulin sensitivity and glucose metabolism.

Sleep and Glucose Regulation

Sleep plays a critical role in glucose metabolism. Poor sleep or insufficient sleep can disrupt your body's ability to regulate blood sugar levels and increase insulin resistance.

Here's how sleep affects glucose metabolism:

- **Insulin Sensitivity:** Sleep is vital for maintaining sensitivity to Insulin. Lack of sleep can reduce insulin sensitivity, leading to higher blood sugar levels.

- **Hormone Regulation:** Sleep also affects the balance of hormones involved in hunger and appetite, such as leptin and ghrelin. Poor sleep can lead to increased appetite, cravings for sugary foods, and overeating, all of which can impact blood sugar levels.

Stress and Blood Sugar

Chronic stress can have a significant impact on glucose metabolism. When you're stressed, your body releases cortisol, the stress hormone, which can raise blood glucose levels by promoting gluconeogenesis in the liver. This means that, even if you aren't eating carbohydrates, the stress response will still raise you blood glucose levels to prepare you to run away from the danger that you feel you are under. This danger could be real, or imagined, either way, the response will be the same!

Stress can also lead to poor eating habits, such as reaching for comfort foods high in sugar and refined carbohydrates, further exacerbating blood sugar imbalances.

Supporting Healthy Glucose Metabolism

Maintaining balanced blood sugar levels is crucial for overall health and well-being. Here are some strategies to support healthy glucose metabolism:

Balanced Diet

Focus on a diet rich in whole, unprocessed foods, including:

- **Whole Grains:** Choose whole grains like oats, quinoa, and brown rice, which have a lower glycaemic index and help maintain steady blood sugar levels.

- **Good Quality Proteins:** Include sources of protein, such as grass fed meat, free range chicken, wild fish, tofu, and legumes, to help stabilise blood sugar and keep you feeling full.

- **Healthy Fats:** Incorporate healthy fats from sources like avocados, nuts, seeds, and olive oil, which can slow the digestion of carbohydrates and prevent blood sugar spikes.

- **Fibre:** High-fibre foods, such as vegetables, fruits, and whole grains, help slow down glucose absorption and improve blood sugar control.

Regular Physical Activity

Aim for at least 150 minutes of moderate-intensity aerobic exercise per week, along with two or more days of resistance training. Regular exercise helps improve insulin sensitivity and supports healthy glucose metabolism.

Prioritise Sleep

Strive for 7-9 hours of quality sleep each night. Establish a regular sleep routine, create a relaxing bedtime environment, and avoid caffeine and heavy meals before bed to improve sleep quality. Poor sleep can have a massive effect on blood sugar.

Stress Management

Incorporate stress-reducing practices into your daily routine, such as mindfulness meditation, deep breathing exercises, yoga, or spending time in nature. Managing stress can help prevent cortisol-induced blood sugar spikes and support overall health.

Symptoms of a Sugar Imbalance

Sugar imbalances, particularly those related to blood glucose levels, can manifest in various ways, affecting energy, mood, and overall health. Identifying and addressing these imbalances is crucial for preventing conditions like insulin resistance, prediabetes, and diabetes. Below are the symptoms associated with sugar imbalances, the recommended tests, and the optimal vs. normal lab reference ranges.

Low Blood Sugar (Hypoglycaemia)

- **Symptoms:**
    1. **Shakiness or Tremors:** Feeling shaky or jittery, especially after missing a meal or after exercise.
    2. **Sweating:** Unexplained sweating, particularly when not related to heat or exercise.
    3. **Hunger:** Intense hunger, often accompanied by cravings for sugary foods.
    4. **Anxiety or Nervousness:** Feeling anxious, nervous, or irritable.
    5. **Dizziness or Light-headedness:** A sensation of spinning or faintness.
    6. **Fatigue:** Sudden tiredness or weakness, particularly after meals.
    7. **Headaches:** Persistent or frequent headaches.
    8. **Confusion or Difficulty Concentrating:** Trouble focusing, thinking clearly, or processing information.
    9. **Blurred Vision:** Difficulty seeing clearly, which may come and go.
    10. **Palpitations:** Irregular or fast heartbeats.

High Blood Sugar (Hyperglycaemia)

Symptoms:

1. **Increased Thirst (Polydipsia):** Excessive thirst, often accompanied by dry mouth.

2. **Frequent Urination (Polyuria):** The need to urinate more often, particularly at night.

3. **Fatigue:** Persistent tiredness or lack of energy, even after a full night's sleep.

4. **Blurred Vision:** Blurry vision that doesn't improve with glasses or contact lenses.

5. **Slow Healing of Wounds:** Cuts or sores that take longer to heal.

6. **Frequent Infections:** Recurrent infections, particularly yeast or urinary tract infections.

7. **Unexplained Weight Loss:** Losing weight without trying, despite eating normally or even more than usual.

8. **Increased Hunger (Polyphagia):** A constant feeling of hunger, even after eating.

9. **Numbness or Tingling in Extremities:** A pins-and-needles sensation, particularly in the hands or feet.

10. **Mood Changes:** Irritability, mood swings, or depression.

Recommended Tests for Sugar Imbalance

Fasting Blood Glucose

- **Purpose:** Measures the concentration of glucose in the blood after an overnight fast.

- **Conventional Lab Range:** 70 to 99 mg/dL or 4-9M mol/L

- **Functional Medicine Optimal Range:** 75 to 85 mg/dL or 4-7 Mmol/L

- **Interpretation:** Levels above the optimal range can indicate insulin resistance or prediabetes, while levels below may suggest hypoglycaemia.

Haemoglobin A1c (HbA1c)

- **Purpose:** Reflects average blood glucose levels over the past 2 to 3 months by measuring the percentage of glycated haemoglobin in the blood.

- **Conventional Lab Range:** 4.8% to 5.6% or 36.6mmol/mol

- **Functional Medicine Optimal Range:** 4.8% to 5.3% or 30-35mmol/mol.

- **Interpretation:** Higher values suggest poor blood sugar control, while values closer to the lower end of the range are optimal for reducing the risk of diabetes-related complications.

Insulin Levels (Fasting Insulin)

- **Purpose:** Measures the amount of insulin in the blood after fasting, helping assess insulin resistance. This can be done as a dried blood spot test as well as a normal blood draw.

- **Conventional Lab Range:** 2.6 to 24.9 µIU/mL

- **Functional Medicine Optimal Range:** 2 to 5 µIU/mL

- **Interpretation:** Higher fasting insulin levels indicate insulin resistance, which can precede the development of type 2 diabetes.

Continuous Glucose Monitoring (CGM)

- **Purpose:** Provides real-time data on blood glucose levels throughout the day and night, offering insights into glucose fluctuations and responses to food, stress, and exercise.

- **Interpretation:** Helps identify patterns of hyperglycaemia or hypoglycaemia and can be used to optimise dietary and lifestyle interventions.

Factors Influencing Blood Sugar Test Results

- **Diet:** Recent carbohydrate intake can significantly impact blood glucose and insulin levels.

- **Stress:** Acute or chronic stress can elevate blood glucose due to increased cortisol levels.

- **Exercise:** Physical activity can lower blood glucose levels, particularly in individuals with insulin sensitivity.

- **Medications:** Drugs like corticosteroids, beta-blockers, and antipsychotics can affect blood glucose levels.

- **Sleep:** Poor sleep or sleep disorders can disrupt glucose metabolism and insulin sensitivity.

- **Hormonal Fluctuations:** Menstrual cycles, pregnancy, and menopause can affect blood sugar levels.

- **Dehydration:** Lack of water intake can concentrate blood glucose and artificially elevate readings.

Supplements to Support you:

Maintaining balanced blood sugar levels is crucial for overall health, particularly in preventing insulin resistance, type 2 diabetes, and related metabolic issues. Along with a healthy diet, low in refined carbohydrates, several supplements have been shown to support blood sugar regulation by improving insulin sensitivity, enhancing glucose metabolism, and reducing inflammation. Here's a list of some of the most effective supplements for helping balance blood sugar:

1. Chromium

- **Role:** Chromium is an essential trace mineral that enhances the action of insulin, improving glucose uptake by cells and supporting stable blood sugar levels.

- **Benefits:** Improves insulin sensitivity, reduces fasting blood glucose levels, and may help reduce cravings for carbohydrates and sugar.

- **Dosage:** 200-1000 mcg per day, typically in the form of chromium picolinate.

2. Magnesium

- **Role:** Magnesium plays a crucial role in glucose metabolism and insulin action. It helps regulate blood sugar levels by improving insulin sensitivity.

- **Benefits:** Lowers fasting blood glucose, reduces insulin resistance, and decreases the risk of developing type 2 diabetes.

- **Dosage:** 200-400mg per day, preferably in the form of magnesium glycinate, citrate, or malate for better absorption.

3. Alpha-Lipoic Acid (ALA)

- **Role:** ALA is a powerful antioxidant that helps enhance insulin sensitivity and glucose uptake in cells. It also protects against oxidative stress, which is often elevated in individuals with blood sugar imbalances.
- **Benefits:** Improves insulin sensitivity, lowers blood sugar levels, and reduces symptoms of diabetic neuropathy.
- **Dosage:** 300-600mg per day.

4. Berberine

- **Role:** Berberine is a compound found in several plants that has been shown to have effects like those of some antidiabetic drugs. It helps to lower blood glucose levels by improving insulin sensitivity and reducing glucose production in the liver.
- **Benefits:** Lowers fasting blood glucose and HbA1c levels, improves insulin sensitivity, and may aid in weight loss.
- **Dosage:** 500mg, 2-3 times per day, taken before meals.

5. Cinnamon

- **Role:** Cinnamon contains compounds that improve insulin sensitivity and slow down the breakdown of carbohydrates in the digestive tract, leading to a more gradual release of glucose into the bloodstream.

- **Benefits:** Lowers fasting blood glucose levels, improves HbA1c, and may reduce LDL cholesterol and triglycerides.
- **Dosage:** 1-6 grams per day of Ceylon cinnamon, or 500 mg of cinnamon extract.

6. Gymnema Sylvestre

- **Role:** Gymnema is an herb traditionally used in Ayurvedic medicine to reduce sugar cravings and regulate blood sugar levels. It may block sugar absorption in the intestines and enhance insulin production.
- **Benefits:** Lowers fasting blood glucose levels, reduces sugar cravings, and may help regenerate pancreatic beta cells.
- **Dosage:** 200-400 mg of Gymnema extract, taken before meals.

7. Inositol (Myo-Inositol and D-Chiro-Inositol)

- **Role:** Inositol, particularly the myo- and D-chiro forms, improves insulin sensitivity and supports healthy ovarian function in women with polycystic ovary syndrome (PCOS), a condition often associated with insulin resistance.

- **Benefits:** Improves insulin sensitivity, lowers blood glucose levels, and may reduce symptoms of PCOS.
- **Dosage:** 2-4 grams per day of myo-inositol or a combination of myo-inositol and D-chiro-inositol in a 40:1 ratio.

8. Omega-3 Fatty Acids

- **Role:** Omega-3s, particularly EPA and DHA found in fish oil, help reduce inflammation and improve insulin sensitivity. They also support cardiovascular health, which is often compromised in individuals with blood sugar imbalances.
- **Benefits:** Reduces fasting blood glucose, lowers triglycerides, and improves insulin sensitivity.
- **Dosage:** 1-3 grams of combined EPA and DHA per day.

9. Vitamin D

- **Role:** Vitamin D plays a significant role in insulin sensitivity and secretion. Deficiency in vitamin D is associated with an increased risk of insulin resistance and type 2 diabetes.

- **Benefits:** Improves insulin sensitivity, supports immune function, and may lower the risk of developing type 2 diabetes.
- **Dosage:** 2,000-5,000 IU per day, depending on blood levels and individual needs.

10. Resveratrol

- **Role:** Resveratrol is a polyphenol found in red wine, grapes, and berries that has been shown to improve insulin sensitivity and support healthy blood sugar levels.
- **Benefits:** Improves insulin sensitivity, lowers fasting blood glucose levels, and reduces oxidative stress.
- **Dosage:** 200-500 mg per day.

11. Probiotics

- **Role:** Probiotics help maintain a healthy gut microbiome, which is increasingly recognized as important for glucose metabolism and insulin sensitivity.
- **Benefits:** Improves insulin sensitivity, reduces inflammation, and may help regulate appetite and weight.

- **Dosage:** A broad-spectrum probiotic supplement containing 10-20 billion CFUs of various strains like Lactobacillus and Bifidobacterium.

12. Bitter Melon

- **Role:** Bitter melon contains compounds that act similarly to insulin, helping to lower blood sugar levels and improve glucose uptake by cells.

- **Benefits:** Reduces fasting and postprandial blood glucose levels, improves HbA1c, and may support weight loss.

- **Dosage:** 500-1000 mg per day of bitter melon extract, or 50-100 ml of the juice.

Conclusion:

Sugar imbalances, whether due to low or high blood glucose, can lead to significant health issues if not properly managed. Recognising the symptoms and using appropriate testing are essential for identifying these imbalances early. Functional medicine practitioners often use narrower, more optimal reference ranges than conventional labs to detect and address imbalances before they develop into more severe conditions. By understanding the factors that influence test results and maintaining glucose levels within optimal ranges, individuals can better manage their blood sugar and overall health.

Supplements can play a significant role in managing and balancing blood sugar levels, especially when combined with a healthy diet, regular exercise, and other lifestyle modifications. However, it is important to work with a healthcare provider to determine the most appropriate supplements and dosages based on individual needs, particularly for those with existing health conditions or those taking medications for blood sugar management.

Glucose metabolism is a complex dance fine tuning hormones, diet, exercise, sleep, and stress. By understanding the factors that influence blood sugar levels and taking proactive steps to maintain balance, you can support your body's energy needs, prevent chronic conditions like diabetes, and promote overall well-being. Remember, small lifestyle changes can have a big impact on your body's ability to manage glucose effectively, helping you maintain steady energy levels and optimal health.

Chapter 7

The Symphony of Female Hormones: Understanding Oestrogen, Progesterone, Testosterone, and More

The female hormonal system is a beautifully complex symphony, where each hormone plays a distinct role in regulating everything from the menstrual cycle and fertility to mood, energy levels, and overall health. So much so, that I consider it one of the "vital signs' that should be assessed by every doctor to ensure that the woman they are assessing is indeed healthy. Vital signs are a group of the most crucial medical signs that indicate the status of the body's vital functions, such as blood pressure, pulse rate, temperature and breathing rate, but in women, any change in her menstrual cycle, any symptoms such as pain or suffering of any kind, is another indication that something is not right with the body's vital functions!

Unfortunately, instead of identifying what is causing the symptoms, such as cramps, migraines, bleeding changes etc, the first line of treatment in conventional medicine is to prescribe a hormone in the form of a pill, patch, IUD or injection. And they may very well remove some of the symptoms (or make them worse), but the cause is not being addressed. The causes are generally sub optimal gut health, unhappy microbiome, nutrient imbalances, stress, poor sleep, compromised detox pathways and a sedentary lifestyle. Identifying these and addressing them accordingly will often fix the problem without the need for any additional hormones. The only time a woman really needs supplemental hormones, is when her body isn't making them anymore. These are discussed in the peri-menopause chapter.

In this chapter, we'll dive deeper into the key hormones that orchestrate these processes, oestrogen, progesterone, testosterone, LH/FSH, and prolactin. Understanding these hormones and how they work together throughout the monthly cycle, can empower you to make informed decisions about your health and well-being. The menstrual cycle is also discussed in more details in the chapter on the fertile years. In this chapter we will touch on the main hormones but remember, they do change over the life span so vary in each life chapter!

Oestrogen: The Feminine Powerhouse

Oestrogen is often considered the primary female hormone, although it's present in both men and women. It's a group of hormones, including estradiol (the most potent form), estrone, and estriol. In women, oestrogen is primarily produced by the ovaries, with smaller amounts being made by the adrenal glands and fat tissues.

The Role of Oestrogen

Oestrogen makes us strong, smart and beautiful and is essential for the development and regulation of the female reproductive system and secondary sexual characteristics. Here's how oestrogen impacts various aspects of health:

- **Reproductive Health:** Oestrogen controls the growth of the uterine lining during the first part of the menstrual cycle, preparing the body for a potential pregnancy. It also regulates the maturation of eggs in the ovaries and supports the growth of breast tissue during puberty. It is also responsible for the growth of breast and hip tissue, giving women their shape.

- **Bone Health:** Oestrogen plays a crucial role in maintaining bone density by inhibiting bone resorption (the breakdown of bone tissue). This is why women are at higher risk for osteoporosis after menopause when oestrogen levels decline.

- **Cardiovascular Health:** Oestrogen has a protective effect on the cardiovascular system by helping to maintain healthy cholesterol levels and supporting the flexibility of blood vessels.

- **Mood and Brain Function:** Oestrogen influences the production of neurotransmitters, such as serotonin, which are involved in mood regulation. This hormone can also impact cognitive function, memory, and overall mental clarity.

- **Skin health**: Oestrogen plays a very important role in skin health, particularly in maintaining skin structure, function, and appearance. Its effects are most noticeable in women, especially during periods of hormonal changes such as puberty, pregnancy, and menopause.

Here's how oestrogen influences skin health specifically:

- **1. Collagen Production**

Collagen is a key protein that provides skin with strength and elasticity. Oestrogen helps stimulate collagen production, which keeps skin firm, smooth, and resilient. As oestrogen levels decline, especially during menopause, collagen production decreases, leading to thinner, sagging skin and the formation of wrinkles.

- **2. Hydration and Moisture Retention**

Oestrogen enhances the skin's ability to retain moisture by increasing the production of natural oils and hyaluronic acid, a molecule that holds water in the skin. This helps keep the skin hydrated, soft, and smooth. When oestrogen levels drop, skin can become drier and more prone to irritation.

- **3. Skin Thickness**

Oestrogen contributes to the maintenance of the skin's thickness by promoting cell turnover and maintaining the integrity of the epidermis (the outer layer of the skin). Thinner skin is more susceptible to damage, bruising, and environmental stressors, which can occur as oestrogen levels decline.

- **4. Wound Healing**

Oestrogen improves skin healing by regulating processes involved in inflammation and tissue repair. Lower oestrogen levels can slow wound healing, which is particularly noticeable in postmenopausal women.

- **5. Sebum Production**

Sebum is the natural oil produced by the skin, which helps maintain moisture and protect against environmental damage. Oestrogen has a balancing effect on sebum production. Higher oestrogen levels during puberty, for instance, may reduce sebum, while lower levels during menopause may contribute to drier skin.

- **6. Pigmentation and Skin Tone**

Oestrogen plays a role in regulating melanin, the pigment that gives skin its colour. During pregnancy or with hormonal changes, fluctuations in oestrogen can lead to hyperpigmentation, such as melasma (dark patches on the face). As oestrogen declines with age, pigmentation changes can also occur.

- **7. Blood Flow and Oxygenation**

Oestrogen helps maintain skin blood flow by promoting the dilation of blood vessels, which ensures good oxygenation and nutrient supply to skin cells. This contributes to a healthy, glowing complexion. A decline in oestrogen can result in reduced blood flow, making the skin appear dull and less vibrant.

- **8. Anti-inflammatory Effects**

Oestrogen exerts anti-inflammatory properties, which helps in reducing skin irritation and redness. It can also protect against inflammatory skin conditions such as acne, rosacea, and eczema.

- **9. Antioxidant Protection**

Oestrogen has antioxidant properties that help neutralise free radicals (unstable molecules that can damage skin cells). By protecting the skin from oxidative stress caused by sun exposure, pollution, and aging, oestrogen helps to slow the skin aging process.

Changes in Oestrogen Levels and Skin Effects

- **Puberty**: During puberty, increased oestrogen levels can result in smoother, clearer skin, however, imbalanced hormones and bad gut health can cause the skin to become inflamed and cause acne.

- **Pregnancy**: Hormonal surges during pregnancy may enhance skin glow but can also lead to pigmentation changes.

- **Peri-menopause:** This is where hormones can fluctuate dramatically each month as the body slowly produces less oestrogen and progesterone. Changes in skin, fine lines and wrinkles and changes in hair texture are common.

- **Menopause**: As oestrogen levels drop during menopause, the skin tends to become thinner, drier, and more prone to wrinkles and sagging due to reduced collagen and moisture.

Oestrogen Imbalance and the effect on overall Health

When oestrogen levels are too high or too low, it can lead to a range of symptoms and health issues:

- **Oestrogen Dominance:** This occurs when there's too much oestrogen relative to progesterone in the body. This isn't because your ovaries are making too much oestrogen, but rather that your body is struggling to remove it, either due to a sluggish liver, or an unhealthy gut, or both! Symptoms can include heavy or irregular periods, breast tenderness, bloating, mood swings, and an increased risk of conditions like PMS, fibroids and endometriosis.

- **Low Oestrogen:** This is common during perimenopause and menopause, leading to symptoms like hot flashes, night sweats, vaginal dryness, mood changes, and increased risk of osteoporosis and heart disease.

Progesterone: The Calming Hormone

Progesterone is another key hormone in the female reproductive system. It's produced primarily by the ovaries after ovulation during the second half of the menstrual cycle, and in smaller amounts by the adrenal glands.

The Role of Progesterone

Progesterone is often referred to as the "calming hormone" because of its role in balancing the effects of oestrogen and promoting a sense of relaxation and well-being. Here's how progesterone supports health:

- **Menstrual Cycle Regulation:** After ovulation, progesterone prepares the uterine lining for a potential pregnancy by making it thicker and more suitable for implantation of a fertilised egg. If pregnancy doesn't occur, progesterone levels drop, leading to menstruation.

- **Pregnancy:** During pregnancy, progesterone is essential for maintaining the uterine lining and preventing contractions that could lead to miscarriage. It also helps the body prepare for breastfeeding by promoting the development of milk-producing glands in the breasts.

- **Mood and Sleep:** Progesterone binds to the GABA receptors in the brain and has a calming effect on the brain and nervous system. It can promote better sleep and reduce anxiety and irritability, especially during the luteal phase of the menstrual cycle (the time between ovulation and menstruation).

Progesterone Imbalance

Imbalances in progesterone levels can lead to various symptoms:

- **Low Progesterone:** Symptoms of low progesterone can include irregular periods, spotting between periods, difficulty conceiving, mood swings, anxiety, and sleep disturbances. Low progesterone is often seen in conditions like polycystic ovary syndrome (PCOS) and during perimenopause.

- **Progesterone Deficiency/Luteal phase defects:** A deficiency in progesterone can lead to oestrogen dominance, where the effects of oestrogen become more pronounced due to a lack of balance. This can contribute to conditions like miscarriage, PMS, heavy periods, and fibroids.

- **Excess Progesterone:** Symptoms of excess progesterone, usually caused by medications or ovarian cysts, include fatigue, bloating, water retention, and breast tenderness, along with psychological symptoms like anger, anxiety or depression.

Testosterone: The Androgen in Women

Testosterone is often thought of as a male hormone (also known as an Androgen), but it's also an important hormone in women. Although women produce much lower levels of testosterone compared to men, it still plays a significant role in health and well-being. Testosterone is actually the precursor hormone for oestrogen, which means, all oestrogen is formed by the action of the enzyme aromatase, on testosterone!

The Role of Testosterone

In women, testosterone is produced by the ovaries, adrenal glands, and peripheral tissues. It serves several important functions:

- **Sex Drive:** Testosterone is a key hormone in regulating libido in women. It helps maintain sexual desire and arousal.

- **Muscle and Bone Strength:** Testosterone contributes to muscle mass and strength, as well as bone density. It helps maintain lean muscle tissue and supports the overall structure of bones.

- **Mood and Energy:** Testosterone can influence mood, energy levels, and motivation. Balanced levels of testosterone contribute to a sense of vitality and well-being.

Testosterone Imbalance

Both high and low levels of testosterone can cause issues in women:

- **High Testosterone:** Although some women have naturally high testosterone, when there are symptoms and the elevated testosterone levels are not her natural state, then consider conditions like PCOS that lead to symptoms such as acne, excess facial or body hair (hirsutism), irregular periods, and difficulty conceiving.

- **Low Testosterone:** Low testosterone levels can result in a reduced sex drive, low energy, decreased muscle mass, and mood disturbances such as depression or a lack of motivation.

LH and FSH: The Cycle Regulators

Luteinizing hormone (LH) and follicle-stimulating hormone (FSH) are critical hormones in the regulation of the menstrual cycle and reproductive health. These hormones are produced by the pituitary gland in the brain and work together to control the functions of the ovaries.

The Role of FSH

FSH is responsible for stimulating the growth and maturation of ovarian follicles (the structures that contain eggs) during the first half of the menstrual cycle. As the follicles develop, they produce oestrogen, which prepares the body for ovulation.

The Role of LH

LH plays a key role in triggering ovulation. Midway through the menstrual cycle, a surge in LH levels causes the mature follicle to release an egg from the ovary, a process known as ovulation. After ovulation, LH supports the formation of the corpus luteum, a temporary structure that produces progesterone to maintain the uterine lining for a potential pregnancy.

LH and FSH Imbalance

Imbalances in LH and FSH levels can lead to menstrual irregularities and fertility issues:

- **High LH/FSH Ratio:** A higher than normal ratio of LH to FSH is often seen in women with PCOS. This imbalance can disrupt ovulation and lead to irregular periods or infertility.

- **Low FSH Levels:** Low levels of FSH can result in insufficient follicle development, leading to irregular or absent periods and difficulties with ovulation and conception.

- **High FSH:** High levels of FSH tend to occurs when the ovaries slow their production of oestrogen during peri menopause. Very high FSH can indicate menopause or premature ovarian failure. Regardless of the cause, it indicates poor fertility.

Prolactin: The Lactation Hormone

Prolactin is a hormone produced by the pituitary gland, primarily known for its role in promoting milk production (lactation) after childbirth. However, prolactin also has other important functions in the body.

The Role of Prolactin

Prolactin is crucial for breastfeeding, as it stimulates the mammary glands in the breasts to produce milk. Beyond its role in lactation, prolactin also influences reproductive health and can affect menstrual cycles:

- **Inhibiting Ovulation:** High levels of prolactin can suppress the release of FSH and LH, leading to a decrease in oestrogen and progesterone production. This is why women who are breastfeeding often experience a natural delay in the return of their menstrual cycles.

- **Mood Regulation:** Prolactin also has an impact on mood and can contribute to the feelings of emotional bonding between a mother and her newborn.

Prolactin Imbalance

Imbalances in prolactin levels can lead to several health issues:

- **Hyperprolactinemia:** This condition occurs when there are abnormally high levels of prolactin in the blood. It can lead to symptoms such as irregular or absent periods, infertility, and, in some cases, the production of breast milk in women who are not pregnant or breastfeeding. Hyperprolactinemia can be caused by factors such as stress, certain medications, or benign pituitary tumours (prolactinomas).

- **Low Prolactin:** Low prolactin levels are less common but can occur and may be associated with a lack of milk production in breastfeeding mothers.

Supporting Hormonal Balance

Maintaining a healthy balance of female hormones is essential for overall well-being. Here are some strategies to support hormonal health:

Nutrition

A nutrient-rich diet can support hormone production and balance:

- **Healthy Fats:** Include sources of healthy fats, such as avocados, nuts, seeds, and olive oil, which are essential for hormone production, particularly oestrogen and progesterone. There is more about seed cycling below.

- **Cruciferous Vegetables:** Foods like broccoli, cauliflower, and Brussels sprouts can support oestrogen metabolism and help maintain hormone balance.

- **Fibre:** A high-fibre diet helps regulate oestrogen levels by promoting the elimination of excess hormones through the digestive system.

- **Phytoestrogens:** Foods rich in phytoestrogens, such as flaxseeds and soy, can help balance oestrogen levels by mimicking the effects of oestrogen in the body.

- **Seed cycling** is a naturopathic practice believed to help balance female hormones throughout the menstrual cycle by incorporating specific seeds into the diet at different phases. Certain seeds contain nutrients and compounds that support the production and metabolism of key hormones, such as oestrogen and progesterone, thus influencing hormone balance over time.

How Seed Cycling Works:

The menstrual cycle is divided into two primary phases: the **follicular phase** (from menstruation to ovulation) and the **luteal** phase (from ovulation to the start of the next period). Seed cycling aligns different seeds with these phases to promote hormonal balance.

1. **Follicular Phase (Day 1–14):**

    - Seeds: **Flaxseeds and pumpkin seeds** (1–2 tablespoons daily)

    - Hormonal Focus: **Oestrogen production**

    - Rationale:

        - **Flaxseeds** contain **lignans**, compounds that have phytoestrogen properties, which can modulate oestrogen levels by binding to oestrogen receptors and influencing oestrogen metabolism. This may help regulate oestrogen levels, especially if they are too high.

        - **Pumpkin seeds** are rich in **zinc**, which is believed to support the production of progesterone later in the cycle.

2. **Luteal Phase (Day 15–28):**

    - Seeds: **Sesame seeds and sunflower seeds** (1–2 tablespoons daily)

    - Hormonal Focus: **Progesterone production**

    - Rationale:

- **Sesame seeds** also contain lignans, which help manage oestrogen levels, and are rich in zinc, important for overall hormone balance.

- **Sunflower seeds** are high in **vitamin E** and **selenium**, nutrients that support the production of progesterone and help detoxify excess oestrogen.

Potential Influence on Hormones:

1. **Oestrogen Regulation**:

- During the follicular phase, lignans in flaxseeds and sesame seeds can help balance oestrogen levels. They may assist the body in managing both low and high oestrogen, supporting a more regulated hormonal environment.

2. **Progesterone Support**:

- In the luteal phase, zinc from pumpkin seeds and vitamin E from sunflower seeds may support the production of progesterone, which is crucial for regulating the menstrual cycle and supporting pregnancy. Balanced progesterone levels are also important for counteracting the effects of excess oestrogen.

3. **Nutrient Support for Hormone Synthesis:**

- Seeds are packed with omega-3 and omega-6 fatty acids, fibre, antioxidants, and essential minerals, which can improve overall reproductive health. These nutrients are involved in hormone production, inflammation control, and detoxification of excess hormones.

Stress Management

Chronic stress can disrupt hormone balance, particularly by increasing cortisol levels, which can interfere with the production of sex hormones. Incorporate stress-reducing practices such as mindfulness, meditation, and regular physical activity into your routine.

Sleep

Quality sleep is essential for hormonal balance. Aim for 7-9 hours of uninterrupted sleep each night, and establish a regular sleep routine to support your body's natural hormone production.

Regular Check-Ups

Regular medical check-ups can help monitor hormone levels and catch any imbalances early. If you're experiencing symptoms of hormone imbalance, such as irregular periods, mood swings, or changes in libido, it's important to consult with a healthcare provider for appropriate testing and treatment.

Testing:

These hormones can be tested in blood, saliva and urine and dried urine tests.

Hormone levels fluctuate throughout the day and vary by individual. That's why it's useful to test oestrogen, progesterone, and testosterone in various ways. Here's a breakdown of the most common methods:

1. **Blood Testing**: This is the most common method and measures the level of "free" and "bound" hormones (those attached to proteins in the blood). It's particularly good for measuring overall hormone levels.

   o **Best for**: Monitoring the total levels of hormones like testosterone and oestrogen in the bloodstream. Often used by doctors to diagnose hormone imbalances.

   o **Timing**: For women, progesterone is best tested about 7 days before the expected period (around day 21 of a 28-day cycle) to check if ovulation occurred. If you want to test your hormones for fertility, then ideally you want to assess day 3or 4 and again on days 19-21 of your cycle.

2. **Saliva Testing**: This measures the amount of "free" hormones — the hormones not bound to proteins and thus available to be used by the body. It gives insight into how much of the hormone is available at the tissue level.

   o **Best for**: Testing the active forms of hormones, such as cortisol, oestrogen, or progesterone. It's commonly used to assess adrenal health and monitor changes over the day.

   o **Timing**: Best for checking hormone levels multiple times during the day (e.g., cortisol) or across a menstrual cycle for women.

3. **Urine Testing**: Urine testing is useful because it can show how your body is metabolising hormones, giving a fuller picture of overall hormonal health. It measures hormone by-products (metabolites) excreted in urine.

   o **Best for**: Understanding hormone metabolism, especially oestrogen. It can indicate if your body is breaking down oestrogen into more protective or harmful by-products.

   o **Timing**: This is often a 24-hour collection, but there's also a more convenient option — dried urine testing.

4. **Dried Urine Testing:** This involves collecting urine samples on strips that dry, which can then be sent for analysis. It's a more comprehensive way to evaluate both hormone levels and metabolism, especially for oestrogen and testosterone.

   o **Best for:** Monitoring hormone metabolites and understanding the balance of various hormone breakdown products. It can also assess adrenal function.

   o **Timing:** Taken throughout the day (4–5 times) on about days 19-21 of the menstrual cycle, capturing fluctuations and giving a detailed snapshot of hormonal rhythms. If your cycle is irregular, you can use LH testing strips (they test for ovulation) and you should test 5-7 days after a positive ovulation results. Another option is a test called Cycle Mapping, where you test your urine every 2 days for a full cycle and the lab can then plot the times where your hormones went up and down through the month. This test is best in women with very irregular cycles, women struggling with fertility or woman who still have their ovaries but have had their uterus removed and thus don't have an obvious menstruation to plot their cycle with.

Best Method to Test Hormone Activity and Metabolism

- **Blood testing** is great for capturing general hormone levels, but it doesn't tell you how your body is using those hormones.

- **Saliva testing** provides a look at active, bioavailable hormones, which can reflect how your tissues are affected.

- **Urine or dried urine testing** is the best way to assess **hormone metabolism**. It shows not only how much of a hormone is in your system but also how it's being processed. For instance, oestrogen is broken down into metabolites that can have protective or harmful effects, and the dried urine test reveals that balance.

Conclusion:

The female hormonal system is a dynamic and interconnected network that requires balance and harmony to function optimally. By understanding the roles of key hormones like oestrogen, progesterone, testosterone, LH/FSH, and prolactin, and how they interact with each other and how they change throughout the month and years, you can take proactive steps to support your hormonal health. Remember, small lifestyle changes, such as eating a balanced diet, managing stress, and prioritising sleep, can have a significant impact on maintaining this delicate balance, promoting not just reproductive health, but overall well-being.

Chapter 8

The Symphony of Male Hormones: Understanding Testosterone, Oestrogen, Progesterone, and More

Just like the female hormonal system, the male hormonal system is a finely tuned symphony, where various hormones play critical roles in maintaining health, vitality, and well-being. Just as with women, the hormones in men are responsible for regulating everything from physical development and reproductive function to mood, energy levels, and overall health. In this chapter, we'll explore the key hormones that orchestrate these processes, testosterone, oestrogen, progesterone, and others. Understanding how these hormones function and interact can provide valuable insights into optimising male health.

Testosterone: The Masculine Powerhouse

Testosterone is often thought of as the quintessential male hormone, although it is present in both men and women. In men, testosterone is primarily produced in the testes, with smaller amounts being produced by the adrenal glands.

The Role of Testosterone

Testosterone is central to many aspects of male health, influencing physical, mental, and emotional well-being:

- **Sexual Development:** Testosterone is crucial during puberty, driving the development of male secondary sexual characteristics such as increased muscle mass, deepening of the voice, and growth of facial and body hair. It also supports the growth and function of male reproductive organs.

- **Libido and Sexual Function:** Testosterone is key to maintaining a healthy libido and normal sexual function. It plays a significant role in sperm production and fertility.

- **Muscle Mass and Strength:** Testosterone promotes the development and maintenance of muscle mass and strength. It helps regulate protein synthesis, which is essential for building and repairing muscle tissue.

- **Bone Density:** Testosterone contributes to maintaining bone density, which helps prevent osteoporosis and fractures as men age.

- **Mood and Cognitive Function:** Balanced testosterone levels are associated with a positive mood, mental clarity, and overall cognitive function. Low testosterone can lead to symptoms such as depression, fatigue, and difficulty concentrating.

Testosterone Imbalance

An imbalance in testosterone levels can lead to a range of health issues:

- **Low Testosterone:** Symptoms of low testosterone can include reduced libido, erectile dysfunction, fatigue, depression, irritability, loss of muscle mass, and increased body fat. Low testosterone can be caused by aging, certain medical conditions, or lifestyle factors such as poor diet, lack of exercise, and chronic stress. Low Testosterone is quickly becoming an issue at an alarming rate thanks to these factors!

- **High Testosterone:** While less common, abnormally high levels of testosterone can lead to aggressive behaviour, irritability, acne, and an increased risk of heart disease. Excess testosterone can also result from the use of anabolic steroids or certain medical conditions.

Assessing Epi-Testosterone

Epi-Testosterone, often simply referred to as Epi-T, is another naturally occurring steroid hormone in your body. It's a close relative of testosterone, although both Epi-Testosterone doesn't have the same muscle-building effects as testosterone, it plays a vital role in maintaining the balance of hormones in your body. It's like a backstage crew member at the musical - you may not see it in the spotlight, but it's working hard behind the scenes to ensure everything runs smoothly. It is best assessed using a dried urine test and is used to assess a true low testosterone reading in the dried urine results.

- **Low urinary Testosterone but normal or high Epi-testosterone:** Epi-testosterone is measured in dried urine tests because in a small percentage of men, who don't convert testosterone into the metabolite that can be analysed in the urine, epi-testosterone, which is made at the same rate as testosterone, is used to confirm whether the low urine testosterone is indeed low, or that it is low due to defect in the UGT enzyme a relatively rare enzyme deficiency, most often seen in people of Asian descent. If the pattern is low testosterone but normal or high epi-testosterone, then a blood test to confirm normal testosterone is recommended.

- If the result is **low testosterone and low epi-testosterone**, this is more indicative of low testosterone but should also be confirmed using a blood test.

- **If testosterone is much higher than epi-testosterone**, then this may indicate an exogenous supply of testosterone is being used.

- **High Epi-T and normal testosterone:** High levels of Epi-T could be a result of external factors like stress, as stress can disrupt your body's hormone balance. It's important to note that while Epi-T is a relative of testosterone, it doesn't have the same muscle-building effects, so high levels won't necessarily lead to increased muscle mass.

Oestrogen: The Surprising Player in Male Health

Oestrogen is typically associated with female health, but it also plays an important role in men. In men, oestrogen is produced in small amounts by converting testosterone into oestradiol, the most active form of oestrogen, through a process called aromatization.

The Role of Oestrogen in Men

Oestrogen is crucial for several physiological functions in men:

- **Bone Health:** Just as in women, oestrogen is essential for maintaining bone density in men. It helps regulate bone remodelling and prevents bone loss, which is critical for preventing osteoporosis as men age.

- **Cardiovascular Health:** Oestrogen has a protective effect on the cardiovascular system by promoting healthy cholesterol levels and supporting the function of blood vessels.

- **Brain Function:** Oestrogen supports cognitive function and emotional well-being. It influences the production of neurotransmitters, such as serotonin, which play a role in mood regulation.

Oestrogen Imbalance

Imbalances in oestrogen levels in men can lead to various health issues:

- **High Oestrogen:** Elevated oestrogen levels in men can result in symptoms such as gynecomastia (the development of breast tissue), reduced libido, erectile dysfunction, and infertility. High oestrogen levels can also contribute to mood disturbances, such as depression and anxiety. This condition can be caused by factors such as obesity, liver disease, or the use of certain medications that up regulate the enzyme Aromatase, that converts testosterone to oestrogen in fatty tissue.

- **Low Oestrogen:** Insufficient oestrogen levels can negatively impact bone density, increasing the risk of osteoporosis. Low oestrogen can also contribute to symptoms such as low libido, fatigue, and mood disturbances.

Progesterone: More Than a Female Hormone

Progesterone is often thought of as a female hormone, but it also plays a role in male health. In men, progesterone is produced in small amounts by the adrenal glands and testes.

The Role of Progesterone

Progesterone serves several important functions in the male body:

- **Precursor to Other Hormones:** Progesterone is a precursor to testosterone and other important hormones, including cortisol. It's essential for maintaining the balance of hormone production in the body.

- **Regulating Oestrogen:** Progesterone helps balance the effects of oestrogen in men. It can prevent the overproduction of oestrogen and support the healthy metabolism of this hormone.

- **Prostate Health:** Progesterone is believed to play a role in maintaining prostate health by counteracting the effects of dihydrotestosterone (DHT), a potent metabolite of testosterone that can contribute to prostate enlargement and cancer.

Progesterone Imbalance

Imbalances in progesterone levels can affect male health in various ways:

- **Low Progesterone:** Low levels of progesterone can lead to an imbalance between testosterone and oestrogen, potentially resulting in symptoms such as low libido, fatigue, and mood changes. It can also contribute to conditions such as benign prostatic hyperplasia (BPH) and prostate cancer.

- **High Progesterone:** Elevated levels of progesterone are less common but can occur as a result of certain medical conditions or the use of progesterone-containing medications. High progesterone levels can lead to symptoms such as decreased libido, weight gain, and mood disturbances.

LH and FSH: The Fertility Regulators

Luteinizing hormone (LH) and follicle-stimulating hormone (FSH) are key hormones in the regulation of male fertility. These hormones are produced by the pituitary gland in the brain and work together to control the function of the testes.

The Role of LH

In men, LH stimulates the production of testosterone by acting on the Leydig cells in the testes. This testosterone is then used to support the production of sperm and maintain male secondary sexual characteristics.

The Role of FSH

FSH is essential for the production of sperm in the testes. It stimulates the Sertoli cells, which support and nourish the developing sperm cells. FSH is crucial for maintaining healthy sperm count and fertility.

LH and FSH Imbalance

Imbalances in LH and FSH levels can lead to reproductive issues:

- **Low LH/FSH Levels:** Low levels of LH and FSH can result in insufficient testosterone production and impaired sperm production, leading to symptoms such as low libido, erectile dysfunction, and infertility.

- **High LH/FSH Levels:** Elevated levels of LH and FSH are often a sign of testicular failure, where the testes are unable to produce adequate amounts of testosterone or sperm. This can occur due to conditions such as Klinefelter syndrome, testicular injury, or chemotherapy.

Prolactin: The Lactation Hormone's Role in Men

Prolactin is a hormone produced by the pituitary gland, primarily known for its role in promoting milk production in women. However, prolactin also has important functions in men.

The Role of Prolactin

In men, prolactin plays a role in reproductive health and overall hormonal balance:

- **Regulating Testosterone:** Prolactin can influence testosterone production. Low levels of prolactin are associated with higher testosterone levels, while high levels of prolactin can suppress testosterone production.

- **Sexual Function:** Elevated prolactin levels can reduce libido and contribute to erectile dysfunction by lowering testosterone levels. Prolactin can also impact sperm production and fertility.

Prolactin Imbalance

Imbalances in prolactin levels can lead to various health issues in men:

- **Hyperprolactinemia:** This condition occurs when there are abnormally high levels of prolactin in the blood. In men, hyperprolactinemia can lead to symptoms such as low libido, erectile dysfunction, infertility, and gynecomastia. Elevated prolactin levels can be caused by factors such as stress, certain medications, or pituitary tumour's (prolactinomas).

- **Low Prolactin:** While less common, low prolactin levels can occur and may be associated with symptoms such as fatigue, low libido, and mood disturbances.

Supporting Hormonal Balance in Men

Maintaining a healthy balance of male hormones is essential for overall health and well-being. Here are some strategies to support hormonal health:

Nutrition

A balanced diet is crucial for supporting hormone production and balance:

- **Healthy Fats:** Include sources of healthy fats, such as avocados, nuts, seeds, and olive oil, which are essential for the production of testosterone and other hormones.

- **Protein:** Adequate protein intake is important for maintaining muscle mass and supporting overall hormonal health. Include lean proteins like chicken, fish, and legumes in your diet.

- **Cruciferous Vegetables:** Foods like broccoli, cauliflower, and Brussels sprouts support the metabolism of oestrogen and help maintain a healthy balance between testosterone and oestrogen.

- **Zinc:** Zinc is an essential mineral for testosterone production. Foods rich in zinc, such as oysters, beef, and pumpkin seeds, can support healthy testosterone levels.

- **Saw Palmetto and Nettle root:** Saw palmetto and nettle root may reduce the breakdown of testosterone into its by-product, dihydrotestosterone (DHT). DHT is a more powerful form of testosterone, which can cause prostate growth in men, and in turn affect urinary function.

Exercise

Regular physical activity, particularly strength training, can help boost testosterone levels and improve overall hormonal balance. Exercise also supports cardiovascular health and mental well-being.

Stress Management

Chronic stress can disrupt hormonal balance, particularly by increasing cortisol levels, which can interfere with testosterone production. Incorporate stress-reducing practices such as mindfulness, meditation, and regular exercise into your routine.

Tribulus terrestris is an adaptogenic medicinal plant that is rich many phytonutrients that support male sexual health. These are compounds with anti-inflammatory, antioxidant and energising action, which can help to improve physical and mental wellbeing. Although it doesn't increase testosterone specifically, Tribulus terrestris may improve libido in men and women.

Sleep

Quality sleep is essential for hormonal balance. Aim for 7-9 hours of uninterrupted sleep each night and establish a regular sleep routine to support your body's natural hormone production.

Regular Check-Ups

Regular medical check-ups can help monitor hormone levels and catch any imbalances early. If you're experiencing symptoms of hormone imbalance, such as low libido, fatigue, or mood changes, it's important to consult with a healthcare provider for appropriate testing and treatment.

Testing:

To accurately assess testosterone levels in men, the most reliable method is a **blood test**. There are different types of testosterone that can be measured, and the timing of the test, type of test, and individual factors all affect the results. Here's a comprehensive breakdown:

1. Types of Testosterone Tests

There are three main types of testosterone measurements typically taken in a blood test:

- **Total Testosterone**: Measures the total amount of testosterone in the blood, including both free and bound testosterone.

- **Free Testosterone**: This measures the testosterone that is not bound to proteins (albumin and sex hormone-binding globulin (SHBG)) and is available for use by the body. Free testosterone makes up only about 2–3% of total testosterone.

- **Bioavailable Testosterone**: This includes free testosterone and testosterone loosely bound to albumin. It represents testosterone that can be easily accessed by tissues.

Total testosterone is usually the first test performed, but **free testosterone** or **bioavailable testosterone** can provide more detail in cases where total testosterone levels are borderline or don't correlate with symptoms.

- **Sex Hormone Binding Globulin (SHBG)**: SHBG binds to testosterone, rendering it inactive. Men with higher

SHBG levels will have lower free testosterone. SHBG levels can be affected by factors like age, liver health, and thyroid function. This is why it's important to measure free or bioavailable testosterone alongside total testosterone in certain cases.

- **Luteinizing Hormone (LH)**: LH stimulates testosterone production. Low LH with low testosterone can indicate secondary hypogonadism.

- **Estradiol**: Since some testosterone is converted to oestrogen, measuring estradiol (a form of oestrogen) can help assess hormone balance, especially in men with symptoms of oestrogen dominance.

- **Prolactin**: Elevated prolactin can suppress testosterone levels and may indicate a pituitary issue.

- **Urine or dried urine testing** is the best way to assess **hormone metabolism**. It shows not only how much of a hormone is in your system but also how it's being processed. For instance, testosterone is broken down into metabolites that can have protective or harmful effects, and the dried urine test reveals that balance.

2. Testing Procedure and Timing

- **Morning Testing**: Testosterone levels fluctuate throughout the day, and they are typically highest in the early morning (between 7 a.m. and 10 a.m.). Therefore, it is important to test testosterone levels during this window for the most accurate results.

- **Multiple Measurements**: Because testosterone levels can vary daily and are influenced by external factors, it's often recommended to take multiple blood tests over a few days to get an accurate average.

Testosterone Replacement Therapy (TRT)

TRT is a medical treatment for men with low testosterone levels, designed to restore levels to a healthy range. While it can offer significant benefits, it also has potential risks and drawbacks. Here's an overview:

Pros of TRT

1. **Improved Energy Levels**

   TRT can help alleviate fatigue and increase overall energy levels.

2. **Enhanced Libido and Sexual Function**

   Restoring testosterone can boost sex drive and improve erectile function.

3. **Increased Muscle Mass and Strength**

   Testosterone plays a key role in muscle development, and TRT can help increase muscle mass and strength with appropriate exercise.

4. **Better Mood and Mental Health**

   Many men report improvements in mood, reduced feelings of depression, and enhanced overall well-being.

5. **Improved Bone Density**

   Testosterone supports bone health, reducing the risk of osteoporosis.

6. **Cognitive Benefits**

   Some men experience improved focus, memory, and mental clarity.

7. **Support for Metabolic Health**

   TRT can help reduce body fat and improve insulin sensitivity, contributing to better metabolic health.

Cons of TRT

1. **Potential Cardiovascular Risks**

   Some studies suggest an increased risk of blood clots, heart attack, or stroke, though evidence is mixed.

2. **Blood clots**

   TRT can increase red blood cell production, which may elevate the risk of blood clots.

3. **Prostate Health Concerns**

   TRT may contribute to prostate enlargement (benign

prostatic hyperplasia) and could potentially exacerbate prostate cancer, though more research is needed.

4. **Infertility**

   TRT can suppress natural testosterone production and sperm production, leading to infertility, which may be irreversible in some cases.

5. **Acne and Skin Issues**

   Some men develop acne or oily skin due to increased androgen levels.

6. **Sleep Apnea**

   TRT might worsen sleep apnea, a condition where breathing stops and starts during sleep.

7. **Cost and Commitment**

   TRT often requires lifelong treatment, regular monitoring, and can be expensive.

8. **Injection or Delivery Method Issues**

   Depending on the method (injections, gels, patches), there may be discomfort, inconvenience, or risk of inconsistent dosing.

Considerations

TRT is not a one-size-fits-all solution and should only be pursued under the guidance of a qualified healthcare provider. Before starting TRT, a thorough evaluation, including blood tests and medical history, is essential to weigh the potential benefits against the risks.

Conclusion:

The male hormonal system is a complex and interconnected network that requires balance and harmony to function optimally. By understanding the roles of key hormones like testosterone, oestrogen, progesterone, LH/FSH, and prolactin, and how they interact with each other, you can take proactive steps to support your hormonal health.

Small lifestyle changes, such as eating a balanced diet, exercising regularly, managing stress, and prioritising sleep, can have a significant impact on maintaining this delicate balance, promoting not just reproductive health, but overall vitality and well-being.

Chapter 9

Steroid Hormone Metabolites: Understanding the Pathways, Genes, Enzymes, and Nutritional Influences

Introduction: The Role of Steroid Hormone Metabolites

As you now know, hormones are the body's chemical messengers, orchestrating a symphony of physiological processes that keep us functioning optimally. Among these hormones, steroid hormones, such as oestrogen, progesterone, testosterone, and cortisol, play pivotal roles in regulating metabolism, immune function, reproductive health, and stress responses. However, the story of steroid hormones doesn't end with their production. These hormones undergo complex metabolic processes in the body, transforming into various metabolites that can have their own biological effects.

This chapter delves into the fascinating world of steroid hormone metabolites, the genetic and enzymatic factors that influence their production, and how specific nutrients can optimise these processes. We'll also explore the different methods for testing steroid hormones metabolites, to help you gain insights into your hormonal health.

The Pathway of Steroid Hormone Metabolism

Steroid hormones are made from cholesterol and are primarily produced in the adrenal glands, ovaries, and testes. Once released into the bloodstream, these hormones travel to target tissues, where they bind to receptors and exert their effects. After their primary function is completed, steroid hormones are metabolised and broken down into inactive or less active forms for elimination from the body. However, sometimes, the metabolites are MORE reactive and can cause health issues. This is why it is so important to assess the metabolites and not just the circulating hormones.

Cholesterol and Hormones: The Starting Point

Cholesterol is a building block. Imagine it as a versatile piece of Lego that can be used to create various structures when other Lego pieces are added to it. In your body, this "Lego block" is the base used to make the all the steroidal hormones, which include important hormones like progesterone, oestrogen, testosterone, and cortisol.

The Steroid Cascade

Imagine a series of waterfalls, where each waterfall represents a step in the production and metabolism (breaking down) of steroid hormones. The steroid cascade begins with cholesterol, which is converted into pregnenolone, then progesterone, and eventually leads to the creation of various steroid hormones, including oestrogen, DHEA, testosterone, and cortisol. The enzymes involved in this complex process can be sped up (up regulated) or slowed down (down regulated) by foods and medication and can be influenced by these if you need to adjust the speed, depending on your results.

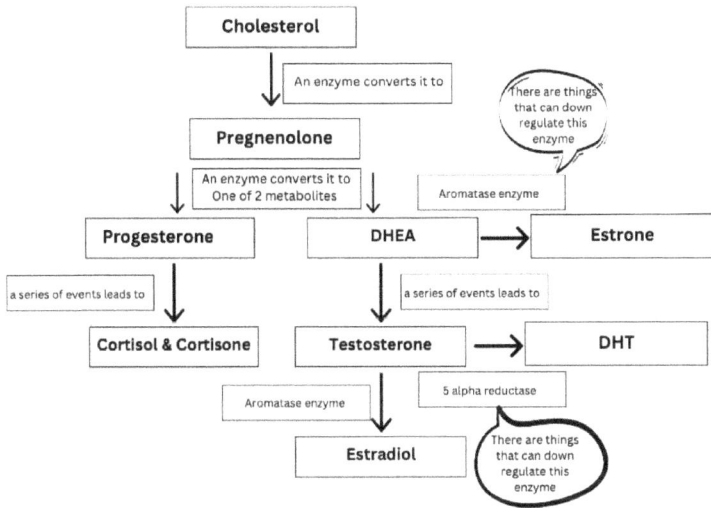

We will start at Progesterone

The first main steroidal hormone that we can assess is Progesterone. Pregnenolone (which isn't assessed in the urine) can be turned into progesterone Or DHEA. Progesterone is a critical precursor hormone, meaning it's a building block to produce other important hormones in the body, especially cortisol!

DHEA

DHEA, short for Dehydroepiandrosterone, is a hormone produced primarily by your adrenal glands from Pregnenolone. It is also made in smaller amounts by the ovaries in women and the testes in men. Like Progesterone, DHEA serves as a precursor, or building block, for the production of other important hormones in the body, particularly sex hormones. DHEA itself has some effects on the body, like influencing mood and energy levels, but its main function is to be converted into other hormones, particularly **testosterone** and **oestrogen**. DHEA is also converted to DHEA(s). If this conversion is low, then it is important to assess inflammation, insulin and the liver.

Cortisol and Cortisone

Known as the "stress hormone," cortisol helps regulate metabolism, blood sugar levels, and the body's response to stress. Progesterone is converted into another hormone called 17-hydroxyprogesterone, which is then used to make cortisol in the adrenal glands. Cortisol is the active stress hormone, but it can also be converted into an inactive form called Cortisone. **Cortisol and Metabolised Cortisol.** Cortisol is metabolised by

5a/5b-reductase (and 3a-HSD) to a/b-THF & THE for excretion. This shows the total amount of cortisol being made (not necessarily used). This process is particularly increased in obesity, high insulin and hyperthyroid, so if you see high metabolised cortisol with low free cortisol, assess these factors. It may be slowed in cases of hypothyroidism, anorexia or poor liver function. So if you see low metabolised cortisol with high free cortisol.

Testosterone

Progesterone is a precursor to androgens, including testosterone, which is essential for male sexual development, muscle mass, and libido. Progesterone is first converted into 17-hydroxyprogesterone, and then further into androstenedione, which can then be converted into testosterone. Don't worry, you don't need to know each step, but the person assessing you should! Testosterone is also an important hormone in women, improving bone health, energy and libido. It breaks down into and potentially more active metabolite called DHT.

Dihydrotestosterone (DHT): Testosterone can be converted into DHT by an enzyme called 5a-Reductase which is increased by high insulin and obesity. DHT is a more potent androgen that plays a key role in male characteristics and reproductive functions. In women who have a fast 5a-Reductase enzyme may have symptoms such as hair loss on the head, growth of hair on the face and acne, symptoms associated with PCOS. In men, high DHT can lead to male pattern hair loss and prostate issues. 5a-Reductase may be decreased by saw palmetto, nettles, pygeum, EGCG from green tea, progesterone, zinc and medications like Finasteride.

Testosterone converts to Oestrogen: The conversion of testosterone to oestrogen is a crucial biochemical process that takes place in both men and women. This conversion is primarily mediated by an enzyme called **aromatase.**

How Testosterone Converts to Oestrogen

1. **The Role of Aromatase**

   - **Aromatase** is an enzyme found in various tissues, including fat tissue, the ovaries, testes, brain, and even in some breast tissues. This enzyme facilitates the conversion of testosterone into **estradiol**, which is the most potent form of oestrogen.

   - The chemical process involves the removal of a methyl group from the testosterone molecule and the formation of an aromatic ring, hence the name "aromatase."

2. **Conversion Pathway**

- **Testosterone → Aromatase → Estradiol**

- This conversion happens in several tissues, but it is particularly active in fat tissue, which is why individuals with higher body fat percentages tend to have higher oestrogen levels.

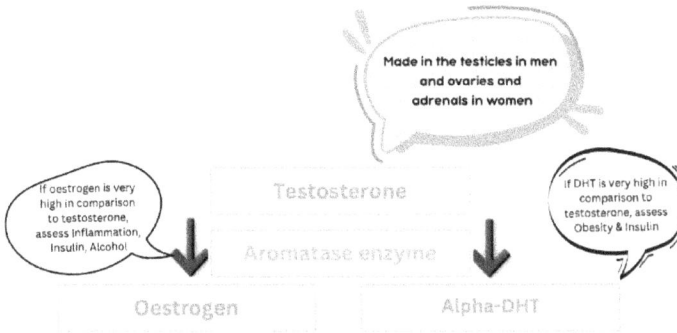

Factors Influencing the Conversion

Several factors influence how much testosterone is converted into oestrogen:

1. **Aromatase Activity**

- The level of aromatase enzyme in the body is a primary factor. Higher levels of aromatase lead to more testosterone being converted into oestrogen. Aromatase is up regulated by insulin resistance and obesity, as well as alcohol consumption. It can be down regulated zinc, flaxseeds, nettles and green tea as well as a low carb diet.

- **Genetics** can play a role in determining how much aromatase your body produces. Some people naturally have higher or lower levels of this enzyme.

2. **Body Fat**

- **Adipose (fat) tissue** has high levels of aromatase. The fatter tissue a person has, the more testosterone can be converted into oestrogen. This is particularly significant in men, where increased body fat can lead to higher oestrogen levels, potentially affecting hormone balance.

3. **Age**

- As people age, especially in men, testosterone levels often decline, and the relative activity of aromatase can increase, leading to higher oestrogen levels.

- In women, the balance shifts during menopause when ovarian oestrogen production drops, but peripheral conversion (from fat tissue) can still maintain some oestrogen levels.

4. **Health Conditions**

- Certain health conditions, like **obesity**, **insulin resistance**, and **polycystic ovary syndrome (PCOS)**, can influence aromatase activity and thus increase oestrogen production.

- **Liver disease** can also impact oestrogen metabolism, as the liver is responsible for processing and breaking down oestrogen. If the liver isn't functioning well, oestrogen levels can rise.

5. **Medications and Substances**

- Some medications, like **anabolic steroids** or **hormone replacement therapy** drugs, can influence the levels of testosterone and oestrogen by either inhibiting or promoting aromatase activity.

- **Alcohol** can increase aromatase activity, leading to higher oestrogen levels.

6. **Inflammation**

   o Chronic inflammation can increase aromatase activity. This is because inflammation often leads to higher levels of certain cytokines, which can stimulate aromatase.

7. Nutritional Factors

- **Diet** and **nutrition** can also influence aromatase activity. For example, diets high in processed foods and sugars can contribute to increased body fat and inflammation, thereby raising aromatase activity.

- Certain compounds found in food, like flavonoids (in fruits and vegetables), can inhibit aromatase activity, potentially reducing the conversion of testosterone to oestrogen.

Oestrogen(s)

Estradiol: Testosterone can be converted into oestradiol, the most potent form of oestrogen. Estradiol is crucial for female reproductive health, including the regulation of the menstrual cycle and pregnancy.

Estrone: Another form of oestrogen that can be produced from androstenedione, which is itself derived from progesterone. Estrone is a weaker oestrogen compared to oestradiol but still plays a role in reproductive health. It is predominantly made after menopause.

Estriol: Estriol is one of three oestrogen hormones. Estriol levels usually rise throughout pregnancy, helping to keep your uterus and unborn baby healthy. The levels are at their highest right before childbirth. They help prepare your body for labour and delivery. Everyone makes estriol. But in people who aren't pregnant, the levels are almost undetectable, unless they have high amount of 16-OH Estrone (discussed on the next page), that can convert to estriol to be removed in the urine.

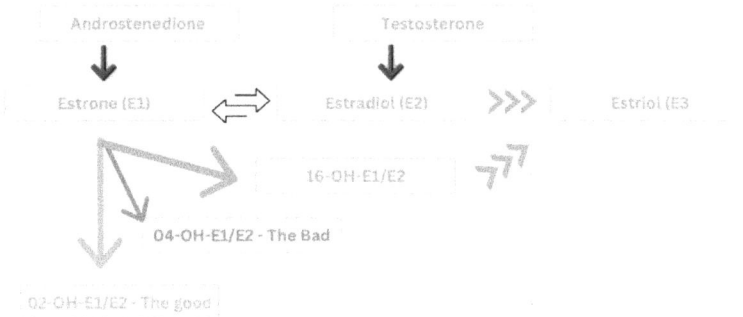

Metabolites Produced in Phase 1

1. **2-Hydroxyestrogens (2-OH) – The Good**

   - **Pros**: These are considered "good" metabolites. They have weak oestrogenic activity and are less likely to cause cellular damage. 2-hydroxyestrone, for instance, is associated with a reduced risk of oestrogen-related cancers, like breast cancer. It is created by the enzyme CYP1A1.

2. **4-Hydroxyestrogens (4-OH) – The Bad**

   - **Cons**: These are considered potentially harmful metabolites. They have stronger oestrogenic activity and can form DNA-damaging compounds, increasing the risk of mutations and potentially leading to cancer. 4-hydroxyestrone is particularly concerning because it can form reactive intermediates that bind to DNA and cause damage. It is created by the enzyme CYP1B1.

3. **16α-Hydroxyestrogens (16α-OH) – The Ugly**

- **Mixed**: 16α-hydroxyestrone is a potent estrogenic metabolite. While it helps maintain bone density and has some protective effects, it can also promote the growth of oestrogen-sensitive tissues, which may contribute to the risk of oestrogen-dependent cancers. This is created by the enzyme CYP3A4.

If your 3 oestrogens and their metabolites are high, you need to assess why!

The 2 main reasons are:

1 – gut health – you may have an enzyme called Beta-Glucuronidase that breaks the bonds created to make oestrogen safe to remove in urine and bile or

2 – your liver needs help

Please check both!

Oestrogen metabolism involves two key phases of detoxification in the liver: **Phase 1** and **Phase 2**. Each phase plays a critical role in breaking down and eliminating oestrogens, but the process can produce both beneficial and harmful metabolites.

Phase 1 Detoxification: Breakdown of Oestrogen

In Phase 1, the liver enzymes known as **cytochrome P450** enzymes metabolise oestrogens, such as estradiol, estrone, and estriol. The goal is to make these hormones more water-soluble so they can be excreted from the body.

Enzymes are like specialised workers that help transform these basic pieces into different hormones. They carefully modify pregnenolone into various hormones, each with a specific role in the body.

These enzymes can work faster or slower in people, depending on genetics, environmental toxins and nutrients. You can see which enzymes are faster or slower in a urine hormone metabolite test. If you see the result of the precursor to the metabolite is low and the metabolite is high, you might need to slow that enzyme down a bit and if you see the precursor to the metabolite is high and the metabolite is low, then you might need to speed up the enzyme. You can do this with a variety of nutrients depending on the enzyme.

The main enzymes that we keep an eye on for safe metabolism of the steroid hormones include the Phase 1 and 2 detoxification enzymes.

CYP1B1 which if upregulated can increase the levels of the more dangerous oestrogen metabolite called 4OH. This enzyme can be slowed down by hops, bioflavonoids and grapefruit.

CYP3A4 creates the metabolite 16OH and if 16OH is higher than ideal, then this enzyme can be downregulated by grapefruit, pomegranate juice, peppermint oil and the herb valerian.

CYP1A1 is the enzyme we want to have the most activity, this creates the more beneficial metabolite 2OH. If the activity of CYP1A1 is slow, it can be improved using cruciferous vegetables. These contain Indole-3-Carbinole which converts to a substance called DIM which improves the activity of this enzyme. I discuss the differences between Indole-3-Carbinole DIM as supplements later in the book.

COMT is the Phase 2 enzyme that along with glutathione, helps to remove bind and remove the phase 1 metabolites. COMT is one of the main methylation enzymes. Methylation of 2-OH/4-OH oestrogens is slowed with certain genetic variants (MTHFR, COMT). If you have slow COMT activity, this can be improved eating cruciferous vegetables and using magnesium supplements and B vitamins.

GST (Glutathione S-Transferase). This enzyme family is involved in the conjugation of glutathione to various steroid hormone metabolites, aiding in their excretion. Variations in GST genes can impact detoxification capacity and influence the risk of hormone-related disorders.

Phase 2 Detoxification: Conjugation

After Phase 1, the metabolites need to be further processed to ensure they are safely eliminated from the body. This is where Phase 2 comes in. Phase 2 detoxification involves **conjugation reactions**, which attach a molecule, such as an amino acid or methyl group, to the metabolites, making them even more water-soluble and ready for excretion.

Key Conjugation Processes in Phase 2

1. ### Glucuronidation

   - An enzyme called **UDP-glucuronosyltransferase (UGT)** attaches glucuronic acid to the oestrogen metabolites. This process makes the metabolites more water-soluble, allowing them to be easily excreted in the urine.

   - **Pros**: Effective at neutralising and eliminating potentially harmful metabolites.

2. ### Sulphation

   - The enzyme **sulfotransferase** adds a sulphate group to the metabolites. Sulphated oestrogens are less active and more easily excreted in the urine or bile.

- **Pros**: Reduces the estrogenic activity of metabolites, helping prevent their reactivation in the body.

3. **Methylation**

   - The enzyme **catechol-O-methyltransferase (COMT)** attaches a methyl group to hydroxylated oestrogens, particularly 2-OH and 4-OH oestrogens.

   - **Pros**: Methylation neutralises potentially harmful metabolites like 4-hydroxyestrone, making them safer and easier to eliminate.

   - **Cons**: If methylation is inefficient, harmful metabolites like 4-OH can build up, increasing the risk of cellular damage.

4. **Glutathione conjugation** is also very important and is discussed on the next page in more detail.

Oestrogen Detoxification:
The Role of Quinone Reductase and Glutathione

Oestrogen detoxification is a critical process that helps maintain hormonal balance and protects the body from harmful oestrogen metabolites. Two key players in this process are **quinone reductase** and **glutathione**. These molecules help neutralize potentially harmful oestrogen metabolites, reducing the risk of DNA damage and related health issues like cancer.

The Role of Quinone Reductase

1. **Quinone Reductase - NAD(P)H - Oxidoreductase 1 or NQO1**

   - Quinone reductase is an enzyme that plays a protective role by reducing the reactive quinone metabolites created by the 4 hydroxy metabolite, back to their less harmful hydroquinone forms.

   - **Reduction Process**: Quinone reductase catalyses the conversion of oestrogen quinones into their less reactive hydroquinone forms. This process helps prevent the quinones from interacting with DNA and causing damage.

   - **Importance**: By neutralising oestrogen quinones, quinone reductase decreases the likelihood of these metabolites forming harmful DNA adducts, thereby reducing the risk of mutations and cancer.

   - **Sulforaphane**: This substance from cruciferous vegetables, but especially broccoli sprouts, can up-regulate this enzyme and is an excellent antioxidant for this very reason.

The Role of Glutathione

1. **Glutathione (GSH)**

   - **Glutathione** is a powerful antioxidant found in nearly every cell in the body. It plays a crucial role in detoxifying harmful substances, including oestrogen quinones.

   - **Conjugation**: In the detoxification process, glutathione is conjugated (attached) to oestrogen quinones through the action of the enzyme **glutathione S-transferase (GST)**. This conjugation process transforms the reactive quinones into more water-soluble, non-toxic forms that can be safely excreted from the body via urine or bile.

   - **Protection**: By conjugating with glutathione, the harmful potential of oestrogen quinones is neutralised, preventing them from damaging DNA or other cellular components.

Factors Influencing Quinone Reductase and Glutathione Activity

Several factors can influence the activity and effectiveness of quinone reductase and glutathione in oestrogen detoxification:

1. **Genetics**

   - Variations in genes encoding quinone reductase (like **NQO1**) and glutathione S-transferase (like **GST** genes) can affect how well these enzymes function. Some people may have genetic variations that lead to lower enzyme activity, making them less efficient at detoxifying harmful oestrogen metabolites.

2. **Diet and Nutrition**

   - **Nutrient-Rich Foods**: Diets rich in cruciferous vegetables (like broccoli, brussels sprouts, and kale), garlic, onions, and foods high in antioxidants can enhance the activity of quinone reductase and boost glutathione levels. These foods contain compounds such as sulforaphane, which can induce the activity of detoxification enzymes.

   - **Glutathione Precursors**: Consuming foods high in sulphur-containing amino acids (like cysteine), minerals such as selenium, as well as vitamins like vitamin C and E, supports glutathione production. Whey protein is also a good source of cysteine, which is a precursor for glutathione synthesis. You can also supplement liposomal glutathione if the need outweighs the body's ability to make its own.

3. **Oxidative Stress**

- **Oxidative Stress**: High levels of oxidative stress can deplete glutathione levels and impair the function of detoxification enzymes like quinone reductase. Oxidative stress can be caused by factors like poor diet, pollution, smoking, alcohol consumption, and chronic inflammation.

- Maintaining antioxidant levels through diet and lifestyle choices is essential for optimal detoxification.

4. **Environmental Toxins**

- Exposure to environmental toxins (like heavy metals, pesticides, and endocrine-disrupting chemicals) can increase the body's demand for glutathione, potentially depleting its levels and reducing detoxification efficiency.

5. **Hormonal Imbalances**

- Hormonal imbalances, such as elevated oestrogen levels, can increase the production of harmful oestrogen metabolites. This increased burden can stress the detoxification system, making adequate quinone reductase and glutathione activity even more critical.

6. **Age and Health Status**

   - ○ **Aging**: As people age, the production of glutathione and the activity of detoxification enzymes tend to decrease, which can reduce the body's ability to effectively neutralise harmful oestrogen metabolites.

   - ○ **Chronic Diseases**: Conditions like liver disease or chronic illnesses can impair detoxification processes, including the function of quinone reductase and glutathione.

To summarise, Oestrogen metabolism involves two key detoxification phases. In Phase 1, oestrogens are broken down into various metabolites, some of which are harmful, like 4-hydroxyestrogens. In Phase 2, these metabolites are conjugated through processes like glucuronidation, sulfation, and methylation, making them safer and more water-soluble for excretion.

Efficient detoxification reduces the risk of harmful oestrogen buildup, while imbalances can increase the risk of oestrogen-related health issues.

Safe vs. Harmful Metabolites

As enzymes work, they can create metabolites that are either safe or potentially harmful. For example:

- **Of Oestrogen - 4-Hydroxyestrogen (4OH)**: A metabolite of oestrogen that can be harmful if it builds up too much, as it might damage cells.

- **Of Oestrogen - 2-Hydroxyestrogen (2OH)**: A metabolite of oestrogen that can be protective, and in its methylated form 2MeOH is very protective! The good news is that with the right foods and supplements, you can pull any excess 4OH down the 2OH route and be safe from any harmful metabolites.

- **Of Testosterone - Dihydrotestosterone (DHT)**: A potent form of testosterone. While DHT is important for things like hair growth, too much of it can lead to problems like hair loss or prostate issues. The good news is, that you can test for this and if your DHT is high, you can use Saw palmetto, Zinc and Nettle to help reduce it.

The balance and activity of these metabolites can have significant implications for health. For example, some oestrogen metabolites are protective, while others may increase the risk of hormone-related cancers.

Nutritional Influences on Steroid Hormone Metabolism Diet and nutrition play a significant role in modulating the activity of the enzymes involved in steroid hormone metabolism. Here are some key nutrients and dietary factors that can influence these pathways:

1. **Cruciferous Vegetables:** Vegetables like broccoli, cauliflower, and Brussels sprouts contain compounds called glucosinolates, which are converted into indole-3-carbinol (I3C) and diindolylmethane (DIM) in the body. These compounds have been shown to support the detoxification of oestrogen by promoting the production of protective oestrogen metabolites (such as 2-OHE1) over harmful ones (such as 4-OHE1).

2. **Methylation Support:** Nutrients that support methylation, such as folate, vitamin B6, B12, betaine (found in beets) and magnesium, are critical for the function of COMT. Adequate intake of these nutrients can help ensure efficient detoxification of catechol oestrogens.

3. **Flavonoids:** Found in foods like citrus fruits, berries, and green tea, flavonoids have been shown to inhibit CYP1B1 activity, potentially reducing the production of harmful oestrogen metabolites. They also support the activity of UGT enzymes, aiding in the clearance of steroid hormones.

4. **Omega-3 Fatty Acids:** Found in fatty fish and flaxseeds, omega-3 fatty acids can reduce inflammation and modulate hormone metabolism. They have been associated with a healthier balance of oestrogen metabolites.

5. **Magnesium:** This mineral is a cofactor for COMT and is essential for efficient oestrogen metabolism. Leafy greens, nuts, and seeds are good sources of magnesium.

6. **Sulforaphane:** A compound found in broccoli sprouts, sulforaphane has been shown to enhance the activity of Phase 2 detoxification enzymes, including those involved in steroid hormone metabolism.

Testing Steroid Hormone Metabolites

Understanding your steroid hormone metabolism can provide valuable insights into your hormonal health and help guide personalized interventions. Several testing methods are available to assess steroid hormone metabolites:

Dried Urine Testing:

- **What it measures:** The dried urine test measures a wide range of hormone metabolites, including those of oestrogen, progesterone, testosterone, DHEA, and cortisol. It provides a detailed assessment of hormone production, metabolism, and excretion.

Other factors affecting the production of primary reproductive and adrenal hormones:

Increased Cortisol: stress, inflammation, Cushing's Disease, obesity

Decreased Cortisol: glucocorticoid use, opioid use, Addison's Disease, Accutane, chronic marijuana use.

Increased DHEA: PCOS, acute stress, Bupropion (Wellbutrin), Alprazolam (Xanax), ADD meds

Decreased DHEA: aging, rapid weight loss, Venlafaxine/Mirtazapine, opioids, glucocorticoids, hormonal birth control, antipsychotic meds, oestrogens, diabetes meds

Increased Testosterone: PCOS, HCG, HGH, L-Dopa, Clomiphene Citrate (Clomid)

Decreased Testosterone: obesity, opioids, hormonal birth control, acute illness, aging, high insulin, steroid use

Increased Oestrogens: PCOS, inflammation, pregnancy, DHEA/testosterone supplementation

Decreased Oestrogens: hormonal birth control, ovarian failure (menopause), opioids, anorexia, underweight

Increased Progesterone: pregnancy, pregnenolone supplementation (increases urine progesterone metabolites, not actual circulating progesterone), Vitex (chaste tree berry)

Decreased Progesterone: hormonal birth control, stress, high insulin, opioids, NSAID use >10 days, anovulation, luteal phase defect, high prolactin, underweight, hypothyroid, hormonal IUD (Mirena)

Conclusion:

Steroid hormone metabolism is a complex process influenced by genetic factors, enzymatic activity, and nutritional intake. By understanding the pathways involved and how to support them through diet and lifestyle choices, you can positively impact your hormonal health and reduce the risk of hormone-related conditions.

Testing your hormone levels and metabolites can provide a clearer picture of your hormonal balance and guide personalized strategies to optimise your health. Whether you assess your hormones nthrough saliva, dried urine, or blood tests, these insights empower you to make informed decisions and take proactive steps toward achieving hormonal harmony.

The results may need a professional who is trained in the reports, to analyse and interpret them.

Regardless of the results, you can affect them positively by nurturing your body with the right nutrients and understanding your unique genetic makeup. You can help your body efficiently metabolise steroid hormones, promoting overall well-being and vitality.

Now that we have covered the basics (and the more complex), let's move on to the life stages and how the hormones can fluctuate and how you can influence them.

Chapter 10

Navigating Puberty: Understanding the Changes, Challenges, and Supportive Strategies for Boys and Girls

Introduction: The Journey Through Puberty

Puberty is a transformative phase of life when children transition into adolescence and eventually adulthood. This period is marked by significant physical, emotional, and psychological changes driven by hormonal shifts. For both boys and girls, puberty brings about a host of new experiences, some exciting, others challenging, as their bodies undergo development and maturation.

In this chapter, we will explore the key changes that boys and girls can expect during puberty, discuss the symptoms of early (precocious) and late puberty, and offer lifestyle and nutritional interventions that can help ease this transition. Understanding these changes and knowing how to support your body during this time can make the journey smoother and less overwhelming.

The Changes of Puberty: What to Expect

Puberty typically begins between the ages of 8 and 14 for girls and between 9 and 16 for boys, although the timing can vary widely. This process is regulated by the hypothalamus and pituitary gland in the brain, which release hormones that trigger the production of sex hormones, oestrogen in girls and testosterone in boys. These hormones are responsible for the physical and emotional changes of puberty. It is important to understand that in the first few years of puberty, the hormones can fluctuate just as much as they do in peri/menopause and it does take a few years for them to settle into their regular cycles.

For Girls:

- **Breast Development:** One of the first signs of puberty in girls is the development of breast buds, which gradually grow into fuller breasts over several years.

- **Menstruation:** Menarche, or the first menstrual period, typically occurs about 2 to 3 years after the onset of breast development. It marks the beginning of a girl's reproductive capability.

- **Growth Spurts:** Girls experience rapid growth in height and weight, often peaking before menstruation begins. The growth spurt usually occurs around ages 10 to 12.

- **Body Hair:** Pubic and underarm hair begin to grow, and some girls may notice hair on their legs and arms becoming thicker.

- **Body Shape:** The body becomes curvier as hips widen, and fat distribution shifts to the breasts, hips, and thighs.

- **Skin Changes:** Increased oil production can lead to acne, especially on the face, back, and chest.

For Boys:

- **Growth of Testicles and Penis:** The first sign of puberty in boys is usually the enlargement of the testicles, followed by the growth of the penis.

- **Voice Changes:** As the larynx grows, boys' voices deepen, sometimes cracking during the transition.

- **Growth Spurts:** Boys typically experience their growth spurt later than girls, often around ages 12 to 15, resulting in a noticeable increase in height and muscle mass.

- **Body Hair:** Boys develop pubic hair, underarm hair, and facial hair, with body hair becoming thicker and more widespread.

- **Muscle Development:** Muscles grow larger and stronger, leading to a more defined, athletic appearance.

- **Skin Changes:** Like girls, boys may experience acne due to increased oil production.

Challenges of Precocious and Delayed Puberty

While most children enter puberty within the expected age range, some experience early or delayed onset, which can present unique challenges.

Precocious Puberty:

- **What It Is:** Precocious puberty is when puberty begins unusually early, before age 8 in girls and before age 9 in boys. This condition leads to the early development of secondary sexual characteristics, such as breast development in girls and testicular enlargement in boys.

- **Symptoms and Impact:** Children with precocious puberty may experience rapid growth initially but may stop growing sooner, resulting in shorter adult stature. They may also face emotional challenges, such as feeling different from their peers or dealing with sexual maturity before they are emotionally ready.

- **Causes:** The exact cause of precocious puberty is often unknown, but it can be linked to certain conditions like brain abnormalities, hormone disorders, or genetic factors. Environmental factors such as exposure to endocrine-disrupting chemicals (found in plastics and some personal care products) may also play a role.

Delayed Puberty:

- **What It Is:** Delayed puberty is when physical signs of puberty appear later than usual—after age 14 in girls and age 16 in boys. It may involve delayed breast development in girls or delayed testicular enlargement in boys.

- **Symptoms and Impact:** Children with delayed puberty may feel self-conscious or anxious about being behind their peers in physical development. They may also be shorter or less physically mature during adolescence, although they typically catch up in height and development eventually.

- **Causes:** Delayed puberty can result from chronic medical conditions (such as coeliac disease or hypothyroidism), nutritional deficiencies, excessive physical activity, or genetic factors. It can also occur in families where late puberty is common.

Lifestyle and Nutritional Interventions to Support Puberty

The journey through puberty can be made smoother with the right lifestyle choices and nutritional support. Here are some strategies to help manage the changes and challenges of this developmental phase:

1. Balanced Nutrition:

- **Protein:** Adequate protein intake is essential for growth and muscle development during puberty. Include good quality meats, poultry, fish, eggs, beans, and legumes in the diet.

- **Magnesium, Calcium and Vitamin D:** These nutrients are crucial for bone growth and density and are especially important before the age of 25 to build up adequate stores in the bones. Encourage the consumption of dairy products, fortified plant milks, leafy greens, and exposure to sunlight for vitamin D. Consider supplementation if needed.

- **Healthy Fats:** Omega-3 fatty acids, found in fish, flaxseeds, and walnuts, support brain development and hormone production. Healthy fats from sources like avocados and olive oil are also important.

- **Iron:** Iron needs increase during puberty, especially for girls starting menstruation. Include iron-rich foods like red meat, poultry, beans, and fortified cereals, along with vitamin C-rich foods to enhance absorption.

- **Fibre:** A diet high in fibre from fruits, vegetables, and whole grains supports digestive health and helps regulate blood sugar levels, which can influence hormonal balance.

2. Regular Physical Activity:

- **Exercise:** Engaging in regular physical activity promotes healthy growth, bone density, and muscle strength. Activities like swimming, cycling, dancing, and team sports also support emotional well-being.

- **Strength Training:** For boys, strength training can help build muscle mass, while for girls, it can enhance bone health and overall fitness. However, exercise should be age-appropriate and supervised to avoid injury.

3. Sleep and Stress Management:

- **Sleep:** Adequate sleep is vital for growth and development during puberty. Aim for 8-10 hours of sleep per night to support physical and mental health. The challenge these days is screen time, which can affect sleep cycles, impact melatonin and have a knock on effect on serotonin and dopamine. Educating your teen on the health impacts of screen time may help them understand and moderate themselves.

- **Stress Reduction:** Puberty can be an emotionally turbulent time. Encourage mindfulness practices, such as yoga or meditation, and ensure a supportive home environment to help manage stress and anxiety. Open communication, be it with a peer, a councillor or someone trustworthy, where they feel comfortable to speak about issues such as bullying and grooming, is also needed these days.

4. Addressing Hormonal Imbalances:

- **Avoid Endocrine Disruptors:** Limit exposure to endocrine-disrupting chemicals by choosing natural or organic personal care products, avoiding plastic containers for food storage, and reducing pesticide exposure by eating organic when possible.

- **Supportive Nutrients:** For girls, omega-3 fatty acids, B vitamins and magnesium can help alleviate menstrual discomfort. For boys, zinc and vitamin D are important for testosterone production.

- **Ensure good gut health:** If any symptoms seem worse than normal, consider assessing the gut. Poor gut microbiome health can contribute to severe acne and other hormonal symptoms during this stage of life.

5. Monitoring Growth and Development:

- **Regular Check-ups:** Routine medical check-ups are essential to monitor growth, development, and overall health. If there are concerns about early or delayed puberty, a healthcare provider can offer guidance and, if necessary, recommend tests or treatments.

6. Emotional Support:

- **Open Communication:** Encourage open conversations about the changes of puberty, providing reassurance and accurate information. This can help children feel more comfortable and less anxious about the changes they are experiencing.

- **Peer Support:** Fostering connections with peers going through similar experiences can help reduce feelings of isolation and boost confidence during puberty.

Conclusion:

Puberty is a time of profound change and growth, shaping not just the body but also the identity and emotional landscape of young individuals. Understanding what to expect and how to navigate this transition with the right support can make a world of difference. Whether dealing with the typical challenges of puberty or facing early or delayed onset, a balanced approach that includes proper nutrition, physical activity, and emotional support is key to ensuring a healthy and positive experience.

As you or your child goes through puberty, remember that this is a natural and essential part of life's journey. With the right tools and understanding, you can embrace these changes with confidence and set the stage for a healthy and fulfilling adolescence and adulthood.

Yes, they may become challenging during this stage, as they try out new versions of themselves to discover who they truly are, but this is all a part of the process and needs love and support so that even if they do "make mistakes" on their journey, they still have a safe space to be themselves.

Chapter 11

Female Hormones in the Fertile Years: Understanding Conditions, Tests, and Nutritional Support

Introduction: The Complex Symphony of Female Hormones

The fertile years, typically spanning from the late teens to the late forties, are marked by a dynamic interplay of hormones that regulate the menstrual cycle, fertility, and overall health in women. This period is not just about reproduction; it is a time when hormonal balance can significantly impact physical, mental, and emotional well-being. Understanding the conditions that affect hormonal health, how to test for imbalances, and the lifestyle and nutritional interventions that can help improve outcomes is crucial for navigating these years with vitality.

This chapter explores common hormonal conditions in women, including fertility challenges, Polycystic Ovary Syndrome (PCOS), Endometriosis, Premenstrual Syndrome (PMS), and Premenstrual Dysphoric Disorder (PMDD). We will discuss the tests available for diagnosing these conditions, the main causes, and the lifestyle and nutritional strategies that can support hormonal balance and overall health.

Whenever thinking about women's health, remember to always look after the G.A.L.S!

Gut: The microbiome both in the gut and vagina, both play pivotal roles in a woman's overall health.

Adrenals: The adrenal glands affect everything, but especially the sex hormones! You can't run away from a tiger AND have a baby; your body will choose survival over reproduction any day!

Liver: Detoxification of hormones or other hormone-like substances should always be supported along with good bile flow and regular bowel movements.

Stress: Well, this is a repeat of the impact of the adrenals, stress affects everything, so make sure that you manage your stress response, find a good therapist, take adaptogens if needed, but get the stress under control or it will control you!

If you look after the GALS, you should have a stress free, symptom free, NORMAL menstrual cycle.

A normal 28-day menstrual cycle is a process that prepares a woman's body for pregnancy each month. It is regulated by the intricate interplay of hormones, which orchestrate various changes in the ovaries and uterus. There are many apps that can track your cycle and will alert you to changes. Here's a detailed breakdown of the phases in a 28-day menstrual cycle:

1. Menstrual Phase (Days 1–5)

This phase marks the **start of the menstrual cycle**. It begins on the first day of menstrual bleeding, which occurs when the lining of the uterus (endometrium) is shed.

- **What happens**: The uterine lining is shed because a pregnancy has not occurred in the previous cycle.

- **Hormone activity**: Oestrogen and progesterone levels are low. This hormonal dip triggers the shedding of the uterine lining.

- **Symptoms**: Women may experience symptoms like cramps (due to uterine contractions), fatigue, and mood changes. Remember that symptoms are not normal, even if they are the norm! Assess your GALS and nutrient needs to make sure you don't suffer. Bleeding usually lasts 3-5 days.

2. Follicular Phase (Days 1–13)

This phase overlaps with the menstrual phase and continues until ovulation. During this time, the body prepares for ovulation by developing ovarian follicles (the sacs that contain eggs).

- **What happens**: Several follicles begin to mature in the ovaries, but typically only one will become dominant and ready for ovulation.

- **Hormone activity**:
  - **Follicle-stimulating hormone (FSH)**: Released by the pituitary gland, FSH stimulates the growth of ovarian follicles.
  - **Oestrogen**: As the follicles grow, they produce oestrogen, which helps thicken the uterine lining to prepare for potential implantation.
- **Symptoms**: Rising oestrogen levels often lead to improved energy, mood, and skin health. There may be light cervical mucus production.

3. Ovulatory Phase (Day 14)

Ovulation occurs around the middle of the cycle, on **day 14** in a 28-day cycle. This is when a mature egg is released from the dominant follicle in the ovary and enters the fallopian tube, where it can be fertilised. I must point out though, that for a variety of reason, women can ovulate well outside this window, so if you are struggling to conceive, please check when you are ovulating using an LH testing kit, available at pharmacies.

- **What happens**: The mature follicle bursts, releasing the egg. The egg can survive for about 12–24 hours, awaiting fertilisation by sperm.

- **Hormone activity**:
  - **Luteinizing hormone (LH)**: A surge in LH (triggered by high oestrogen levels) prompts ovulation.
  - **Oestrogen**: Peaks right before ovulation, helping the uterine lining thicken and become more hospitable to a fertilised egg.
- **Symptoms**: Some women experience mild cramping or twinges (known as mittelschmerz) on one side of the abdomen. Cervical mucus becomes clear, stretchy, and more abundant (often compared to raw egg whites), signalling high fertility.

4. Luteal Phase (Days 15–28)

The luteal phase is the second half of the cycle, after ovulation, and lasts around 14 days. During this phase, the body prepares for either pregnancy or the start of a new cycle.

- **What happens**:
  - After ovulation, the follicle that released the egg transforms into the **corpus luteum**, which produces progesterone to maintain the uterine lining.
  - If fertilisation does not occur, the corpus luteum breaks down after about 10–14 days, leading to a drop in progesterone levels.

- **Hormone activity**:

  - **Progesterone**: Produced by the corpus luteum, progesterone stabilises and thickens the uterine lining for potential implantation.

  - **Oestrogen**: After its peak during ovulation, oestrogen levels slightly drop but then rise again along with progesterone to maintain the uterine lining.

  - If the egg is not fertilised, both progesterone and oestrogen levels fall, triggering the start of the next menstrual cycle.

- **Symptoms**: In the second half of the luteal phase (around days 21–28), many women experience **premenstrual syndrome (PMS)**, which can include bloating, breast tenderness, mood swings, fatigue, and irritability. Cervical mucus dries up and becomes less noticeable as progesterone dominates. Symptoms are a sign that your body needs something; something removed or added. Assess and find out what that may be and you'll be amazed how you can actually be symptom free!

Summary of the 28-Day Menstrual Cycle Phases

Phase	Days	Key Hormones	Main Events
Menstrual Phase	1–5	Low oestrogen, low progesterone	Shedding of the uterine lining (menstrual bleeding)
Follicular Phase	1–13	FSH, rising oestrogen	Follicle development, thickening of the uterine lining
Ovulatory Phase	14	LH surge, peak oestrogen	Release of the mature egg (ovulation)
Luteal Phase	15–28	Progesterone, moderate oestrogen	Corpus luteum formation, uterine lining maintained or shed

Normal cycle pattern:

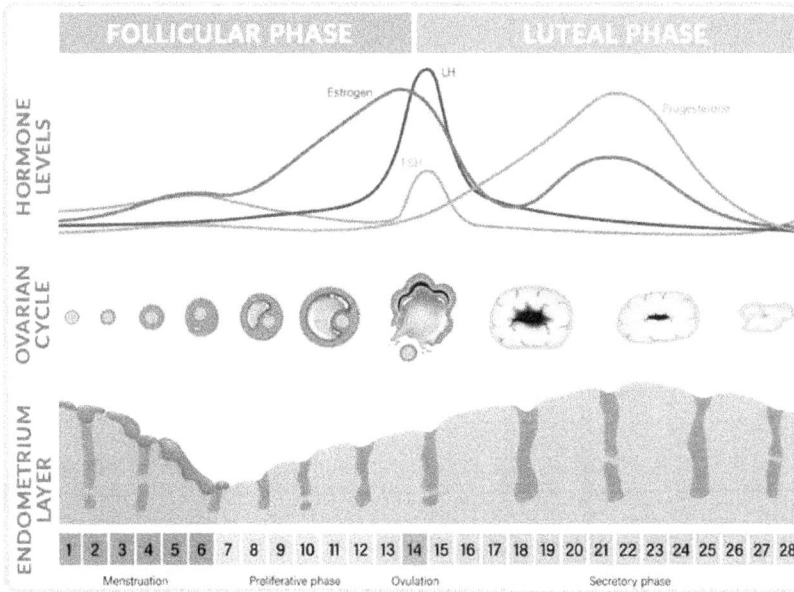

Menstrual Cycle

Surprising benefits to Menstruation!

Menstruation should be looked at as a blessing. It is one of the best ways to reduce the amount of forever chemicals (POPs) that you may have been exposed to. So, every time you have your monthly bleed, you are becoming less toxic and that should be celebrated!

Another exciting development with respect to health and menstrual blood, is menstrual blood banking. Menstrual blood banking is the process of collecting and storing menstrual blood stem cells for potential future use. The stem cells in menstrual blood have similar regenerative properties to those in bone marrow and umbilical cord blood. Menstrual blood banking allows women to preserve their stem cells for their own use or for a family member. Research suggests that menstrual blood stem cells may be used to treat a variety of conditions, including atherosclerosis, diabetes, stroke, rheumatoid arthritis, Parkinson disease, Alzheimer's disease, liver failure, and spinal cord injury. This is exciting stuff! Now let's go back to explaining the hormones, what may go wrong and what you can do about it.

Key Hormonal Conditions During the Fertile Years

1. **Fertility Challenges:**

   - **Overview:** Fertility can be influenced by a variety of factors, including hormonal imbalances, lifestyle choices, and underlying medical conditions. The hormones primarily involved in fertility are oestrogen, progesterone, luteinizing hormone (LH), and follicle-stimulating hormone (FSH).

   - **Symptoms:** Difficulty conceiving, miscarriages, irregular menstrual cycles, and hormonal imbalances detected through blood tests.

   - **Causes:** Common causes include ovulatory disorders, tubal factors, uterine abnormalities, and male factor infertility. Stress and toxicity are also common causes.

- **Testing:** Blood tests to measure hormone levels (e.g., FSH, LH, oestradiol, progesterone), ovulation tracking, and imaging tests like ultrasounds to assess ovarian and uterine health. Cycle mapping tests (dried urine) will detect a luteal phase defect, where progesterone is not strong enough to support a pregnancy.

- **Lifestyle Interventions:** Maintaining a healthy weight, managing stress, avoiding smoking and excessive alcohol, and engaging in regular physical activity can improve fertility outcomes.

- **Nutritional Support:** A diet rich in antioxidants, Vitamin C, beta carotene, omega-3 fatty acids, and nutrients like folate, zinc, and vitamin D can support reproductive health. Supplements such as CoQ10 and inositol may also enhance fertility.

2. **Polycystic Ovary Syndrome (PCOS):**

- **Overview:** PCOS is a common hormonal disorder characterised by irregular menstrual cycles, high levels of androgens (male hormones), and the presence of multiple ovarian cysts seen on an ultrasound. It can affect fertility and increase the risk of other health issues.

- **Symptoms:** Irregular periods, acne, excessive hair growth (hirsutism), weight gain, and insulin resistance. But read more below.

- **Causes:** The exact cause of PCOS is unknown, but it is believed to involve a combination of genetic and environmental factors. Stress, Insulin resistance and inflammation are also implicated, along with excess androgens (testosterone and DHEA).

- **Testing:** Blood tests to measure levels of androgens, insulin, and glucose; pelvic ultrasound to check for ovarian cysts; and hormone testing to assess FSH and LH levels. Assessing the health of the adrenals is also advised.

- **Lifestyle Interventions:** Weight management through diet and exercise is crucial for managing PCOS symptoms. Stress reduction techniques like yoga and meditation can also be beneficial.

- **Nutritional Support:** A low-glycaemic diet rich in whole foods, fibre, and healthy fats can help regulate blood sugar levels. Nutrients like myo-inositol, chromium, and omega-3 fatty acids can support hormonal balance and reduce inflammation. Adaptogens can help if the adrenals are a contributing factor. If the Androgens (testosterone and DHT) are causing symptoms such as hair growth on the face, then spearmint, nettle and saw palmetto can help.

Polycystic Ovary Syndrome (PCOS) can present in various ways, and researchers generally classify the condition into four different phenotypes based on the presence or absence of three main features: hyperandrogenism (excess male hormones), ovulatory dysfunction (irregular or absent periods), and polycystic ovaries on ultrasound.

The four phenotypes of PCOS are:

1. Phenotype A: Classic PCOS (Hyperandrogenism + Ovulatory Dysfunction + Polycystic Ovaries) This is the most common and severe form of PCOS, characterised by:

- **Hyperandrogenism:** Signs like hirsutism (excessive hair growth), acne, or elevated androgen (DHEA and testosterone) levels in blood or urine metabolite tests.

- **Ovulatory Dysfunction:** Irregular or absent menstrual cycles.

- **Polycystic Ovaries:** Multiple small follicles (cysts) on the ovaries seen via ultrasound.

2. Phenotype B: Hyperandrogenism + Ovulatory Dysfunction (But no Polycystic Ovaries)

- **Hyperandrogenism:** Excessive hair growth, acne, or high blood androgen levels.

- **Ovulatory Dysfunction:** Irregular or absent periods.

- **No polycystic ovaries** visible on ultrasound.

3. Phenotype C: Hyperandrogenism + Polycystic Ovaries (But Regular Ovulation)

- **Hyperandrogenism:** Signs of excess male hormones, such as hirsutism or acne.

- **Polycystic Ovaries** on ultrasound.

- **Normal Ovulation:** Regular menstrual cycles and ovulation.

4. Phenotype D: Ovulatory Dysfunction + Polycystic Ovaries (But No Hyperandrogenism)

- **Ovulatory Dysfunction:** Irregular or absent periods.
- **Polycystic Ovaries** on ultrasound.
- **No Hyperandrogenism:** No signs of excess male hormones, such as acne or hirsutism.

Summary of the Four Phenotypes:

- **Phenotype A (Classic PCOS):** Hyperandrogenism + Ovulatory Dysfunction + Polycystic Ovaries.
- **Phenotype B:** Hyperandrogenism + Ovulatory Dysfunction (No Polycystic Ovaries).
- **Phenotype C:** Hyperandrogenism + Polycystic Ovaries (Normal Ovulation).
- **Phenotype D:** Ovulatory Dysfunction + Polycystic Ovaries (No Hyperandrogenism).

Each phenotype has different implications for health, including metabolic risks like insulin resistance, obesity, and cardiovascular disease, and may require different management strategies. No matter which phenotype is presenting, always check insulin, androgens, adrenals and inflammation and work on the root cause with your healthcare provider.

3. **Endometriosis:**

- **Overview:** Endometriosis is a condition where tissue similar to the lining of the uterus grows outside the uterus, usually in the gut, but can grow elsewhere in the abdomen and even the lungs. This causes significant pain in those areas during menstruation as those cells will also bleed. Endometriosis can also potentially affect fertility.

- **Symptoms:** Severe menstrual cramps, chronic pelvic pain, pain during intercourse, heavy periods, and infertility.

- **Causes:** The exact cause of endometriosis is unclear, but it may involve retrograde menstruation, immune system dysfunction, or genetic factors. Other factors that have been attributed to the triggering of endometriosis include copper/zinc imbalance and the presence of an oral bacteria called *Fusobacterium* in the colon. This is why it is important to assess nutrients and gut health if you suspect endometriosis.

- **Testing:** Diagnosis is often made through a combination of pelvic exams, imaging tests like ultrasounds or MRIs, and laparoscopic surgery.

Nutritional testing and a stool test will help identify the potential root causes.

- **Lifestyle Interventions:** Regular exercise, stress management, and techniques like acupuncture may help manage symptoms. Avoiding environmental toxins that can disrupt hormone function is also recommended. Improving the zinc/copper balance and gut health can also help.

- **Nutritional Support:** An anti-inflammatory diet rich in fruits, vegetables, and omega-3 fatty acids can help reduce pain and inflammation. Supplements such as curcumin, omega-3s, B vitamins and magnesium may also provide relief. **Other supplements:** Indole-3-carbinole, DIM and Calcium-D-Glucarate can all be used to ease the symptoms of oestrogen dominance if that is identified as the cause of the symptoms.

4. **Premenstrual Syndrome (PMS) and Premenstrual Dysphoric Disorder (PMDD):**
   - **Overview:** PMS refers to a range of emotional and physical symptoms that occur in the luteal phase of the menstrual cycle. PMDD is a more severe form of

PMS, characterised by extreme mood swings, irritability, and depression.

- **Symptoms:** PMS symptoms include bloating, breast tenderness, lower abdominal pain, migraines, mood swings, fatigue, and headaches. PMDD includes severe mood disturbances, depression, anxiety, and irritability.

- **Causes:** Hormonal fluctuations, particularly changes in progesterone and oestrogen levels, are thought to trigger PMS and PMDD. Neurotransmitter imbalances, such as low serotonin levels, may also play a role. Consider the zinc/copper balance and always assess gut health in these conditions.

- **Testing:** Diagnosis is primarily based on symptom tracking and medical history. Hormone testing may be conducted to rule out other conditions.

- **Lifestyle Interventions:** Regular exercise, adequate sleep, and stress management are crucial. Cognitive-behavioural therapy (CBT) can also be effective for managing PMDD.

- **Nutritional Support:** A diet rich in complex carbohydrates, fibre, and lean proteins can help stabilise blood sugar levels and mood. Calcium, magnesium, and vitamin B6 supplements are often recommended for PMS. For PMDD, omega-3 fatty acids, and herbal supplements like chasteberry may help alleviate symptoms. **Other supplements:** Indole-3-carbinole, DIM and Calcium-D-Glucarate can all be used to ease the symptoms of oestrogen dominance

Gallstones: a common issue in fertile females

Gallstones are more common in women later in their fertile years but are common and avoidable. The hormones oestrogen and progesterone play key roles in the formation of gallstones, especially cholesterol-based gallstones, which are the most common type. Here's how they contribute and how gallstone formation can be prevented:

1. Role of Female Hormones in Gallstone Formation

a. Oestrogen

- **Increases Cholesterol Secretion into Bile**: Oestrogen increases the liver's secretion of cholesterol into bile, a digestive fluid stored in the gallbladder. When too much cholesterol is present, it can precipitate and form solid particles, leading to gallstone formation.

- **Slows Gallbladder Emptying**: Oestrogen also slows down the contraction of the gallbladder, causing bile to sit in the gallbladder for longer periods. Stagnant bile can contribute to the formation of gallstones.

- **Influence During Fertile Years**: Oestrogen levels are higher during a woman's reproductive years, especially during pregnancy and with the use of hormonal birth control or hormone replacement therapy (HRT), which increases the risk of gallstone formation.

b. Progesterone

- **Relaxes Smooth Muscle**: Progesterone, another hormone that rises during the menstrual cycle and pregnancy, relaxes smooth muscles, including those in the gallbladder. This leads to slower gallbladder contractions, resulting in less frequent emptying of bile.

- **Bile Stasis**: This reduced gallbladder motility can lead to bile stasis (stagnation of bile), further increasing the risk of gallstone formation, as bile that sits too long in the gallbladder becomes more concentrated and prone to forming stones.

2. Risk Factors for Gallstones in Women

- **Pregnancy**: High levels of oestrogen and progesterone during pregnancy increase the risk of gallstone formation due to increased cholesterol in bile and reduced gallbladder motility.

- **Hormonal Contraceptives or HRT**: Birth control pills and HRT raise oestrogen levels, which can similarly increase cholesterol secretion into bile and promote gallstone formation.

- **Obesity**: Excess body fat can increase oestrogen levels, even in women who are not pregnant or taking hormone therapy, raising the risk of gallstones.

3. Preventing Gallstones During Fertile Years

To prevent gallstones, especially for women in their reproductive years when hormone levels are naturally higher, several lifestyle changes and preventive measures can be helpful:

a. Maintain a Healthy Diet

- **Fibre-Rich Foods**: Eat a diet rich in fibre from fruits, vegetables, and whole grains to promote healthy digestion and reduce cholesterol levels in bile.

- **Healthy Fats**: Consume healthy fats (e.g., olive oil, avocados, nuts) in moderation. These fats can help stimulate regular gallbladder emptying.

- **Moderate Saturated Fat Intake**: Reducing intake of foods high in saturated fats (like fried or fatty foods) can help prevent cholesterol build-up in the bile.

- **Limit Refined Carbs and Sugars**: High sugar and refined carbohydrate intake can increase cholesterol levels in bile, raising the risk of gallstone formation. Limit processed foods and sugary snacks.

b. Maintain a Healthy Weight

- **Avoid Rapid Weight Loss**: While maintaining a healthy weight can reduce gallstone risk, rapid weight loss can actually increase the risk because it causes the liver to release more cholesterol into bile. Aim for gradual weight loss if needed.

- **Regular Exercise**: Staying physically active can help maintain a healthy weight and improve digestion, reducing the likelihood of gallstone formation.

c. Considerations with Hormonal Contraceptives

- **Alternative Contraception**: Women at higher risk for gallstones (e.g., family history of gallstones or obesity) may consider non-hormonal birth control methods, as hormonal contraceptives containing oestrogen can increase the risk of gallstone formation.

d. Hydration

- **Stay Well Hydrated**: Drinking enough water helps ensure that bile stays fluid and less concentrated, reducing the risk of gallstone formation.

e. Manage Risk Factors

- **Monitor Oestrogen Therapy**: Women taking oestrogen (through HRT or birth control) should consult their healthcare provider about their risk for gallstones and whether adjustments to their therapy are needed.

- **Diabetes and Metabolic Syndrome Management**: Conditions like insulin resistance or metabolic syndrome increase the risk of gallstones, so managing blood sugar and improving overall metabolic health can reduce this risk.

Summary of gallstones:

- **Oestrogen** increases cholesterol secretion into bile and slows gallbladder emptying, raising the risk of gallstones, especially during pregnancy and with the use of hormonal contraceptives.

- **Progesterone** slows gallbladder emptying further, increasing the chance of bile stasis and gallstone formation.

- To prevent gallstones during the fertile years, maintaining a healthy diet, avoiding rapid weight loss, staying active, staying hydrated, and managing hormonal contraceptive use can help reduce the risk.

Cholagogues to the Rescue

Cholagogues are substances that promote the discharge of bile from the gallbladder into the small intestine. Bile is essential for the digestion and absorption of fats. By encouraging the flow of bile, cholagogues help prevent bile stagnation, which is a common factor in gallstone formation.

1. How Cholagogues Work to Prevent Gallstones

Gallstones form when bile becomes too concentrated or stagnant, often due to excess cholesterol or bile salts. Cholagogues help prevent this by:

- **Stimulating Gallbladder Contraction**: This prevents bile from becoming stagnant and too concentrated, which can lead to the formation of cholesterol crystals and eventually gallstones.

- **Enhancing Bile Flow**: By increasing bile flow, cholagogues help keep bile fluid and reduce the chances of solid particles forming.

- **Supporting Digestion**: Improved bile flow helps in the digestion of fats, which can also reduce cholesterol levels in bile, further lowering the risk of stone formation.

2. Natural Cholagogues and Their Role

There are several natural substances and herbs considered cholagogues that may help maintain gallbladder health and prevent gallstones:

a. Dandelion (Taraxacum officinale)

- **Cholagogue Action**: Dandelion stimulates bile production and encourages bile release from the gallbladder. It also supports liver function, helping the liver produce bile more efficiently.

- **How to Use**: Dandelion root can be consumed as tea, in tinctures, or as supplements. Drinking dandelion tea regularly can promote healthy bile flow and reduce the risk of bile stagnation.

b. Milk Thistle (Silybum marianum)

- **Cholagogue Action**: Milk thistle enhances bile production and flow, while also supporting liver health. Its active compound, **silymarin**, protects liver cells and encourages efficient bile production.

- **How to Use**: Milk thistle can be taken in capsule, tincture, or tea form. It's commonly used as a liver tonic but also has gallbladder-supportive properties.

c. Turmeric (Curcuma longa)

- **Cholagogue Action**: Turmeric stimulates the gallbladder to release bile, which aids in fat digestion and prevents bile from becoming too thick and prone to forming gallstones.

- **How to Use**: Turmeric can be added to food, taken as a supplement, or used in teas. Curcumin, the active compound in turmeric, is available in concentrated supplement form.

d. Artichoke (Cynara scolymus)

- **Cholagogue Action**: Artichoke is known to increase bile production and enhance gallbladder function. It also helps lower cholesterol levels in bile, reducing the risk of cholesterol-based gallstones.

- **How to Use**: Artichoke leaf extract is available in supplements or as tea. Consuming artichokes regularly can also support bile flow.

e. Peppermint (Mentha piperita)

- **Cholagogue Action**: Peppermint has been shown to stimulate bile flow and reduce spasms in the bile ducts, helping bile move more freely.

- **How to Use**: Peppermint tea is a simple and effective way to promote bile flow, or peppermint oil capsules can be taken.

3. Dietary and Lifestyle Approaches for Using Cholagogues

Incorporating cholagogues into your diet and lifestyle can help maintain gallbladder health and prevent gallstones:

- **Eat Bitter Foods**: Many bitter-tasting foods act as natural cholagogues. Examples include dandelion greens, radicchio, and arugula/rocket. These can be incorporated into salads and meals to stimulate bile flow.

- **Use Herbal Teas**: Drinking teas made from cholagogue herbs like dandelion, peppermint, or turmeric can be a simple daily routine to support gallbladder health.

- **Cook with Cholagogue Herbs**: Adding turmeric or artichokes to your meals not only provides health benefits but also encourages bile flow.

- **Stay Active**: Regular physical activity helps improve digestion and bile flow, reducing the risk of gallstone formation.

4. Precautions When Using Cholagogues

While cholagogues can be helpful in preventing gallstones, there are some important precautions:

- **Existing Gallstones**: If you already have gallstones, using strong cholagogues could potentially cause the stones to move and block the bile duct, leading to pain or complications. Always consult a healthcare provider before using cholagogues if gallstones are present.

- **Bile Duct Obstruction**: If there's a blockage in the bile ducts, stimulating bile flow can worsen symptoms. Seek medical advice before using cholagogues in such cases.

Understanding Fibroids: Hormonal Influence and Treatment

Fibroids, medically known as uterine leiomyomas, are noncancerous growths that develop within or on the muscular walls of the uterus. They vary significantly in size, ranging from microscopic nodules to large masses that can distort the uterine shape. Fibroids are among the most common gynaecological conditions, affecting up to 70-80% of women during their reproductive years. While some women may remain asymptomatic, others experience significant symptoms such as heavy menstrual bleeding, pelvic pain, and pressure on surrounding organs. Fibroids can negatively impact fertility.

The Role of Hormones in Fibroid Development and Growth

Hormones, particularly oestrogen and progesterone, play a critical role in the development and growth of fibroids. These steroid hormones promote the proliferation of uterine tissue and are believed to stimulate fibroid growth through several mechanisms:

1. **Oestrogen's Impact:**

    o Oestrogen and oestrogenic compounds can promote the growth of fibroids by stimulating cell proliferation and enhancing the production of collagen, a major component of fibroid tissue.

    o Fibroids contain more oestrogen receptors than normal uterine tissue, making them highly sensitive to oestrogen's effects.

    o Higher levels of circulating oestrogen, such as during pregnancy or with hormonal therapies, often result in fibroid enlargement.

2. **Progesterone's Contribution:**

    o Progesterone, while typically associated with stabilising uterine growth, paradoxically supports fibroid expansion by increasing the expression of growth factors and inhibiting cellular apoptosis (programmed cell death).

o   Like oestrogen, fibroids also have an increased number of progesterone receptors, which is why some get worse when treated using progesterone.

3. **Hormonal Fluctuations:**

    o   Fibroids are most prevalent and active during a woman's reproductive years, as hormone levels are high.

    o   Postmenopausal women, who experience a natural decline in oestrogen and progesterone, often see a reduction in fibroid size and symptoms.

4. **Other Factors:**

    o   While oestrogen and progesterone are key drivers, genetic predispositions (women of afro Caribbean decent are more prone to fibroids), growth factors, toxin exposures and local inflammatory changes in the uterus also play a role in fibroid pathogenesis.

Common Symptoms of Fibroids

- Heavy or Prolonged Menstrual Bleeding: Often with clots and can lead to iron deficiency anaemia.

- Pelvic Pain or Pressure: Due to the size and location of the fibroids.

- Frequent Urination or Constipation: Caused by fibroid pressure on the bladder or rectum.

- **Reproductive Challenges:** Including infertility, miscarriage, or complications during pregnancy.

Treatment Approaches

The management of fibroids depends on factors such as symptom severity, size and location of the fibroids, the patient's age, and whether fertility preservation is a concern. Treatments range from conservative measures to surgical interventions.

1. Medical Management

- **Hormonal Therapies:**

    o GnRH Agonists: Medications like leuprolide temporarily reduce oestrogen and progesterone production, shrinking fibroids. These are often used preoperatively or to manage severe symptoms but are not suitable for long-term use due to side effects like bone loss.

    o Progestin-Containing Therapies: Devices like the levonorgestrel-releasing intrauterine system (IUD), often the Mirena coil, can control heavy bleeding, but in some women, this can make the fibroids worse.

- o Selective Progesterone Receptor Modulators (SPRMs): Medications like ulipristal acetate can shrink fibroids and alleviate symptoms.
- Tranexamic Acid: A non-hormonal option to reduce heavy menstrual bleeding.

2. Minimally Invasive Procedures

- o Ablation Techniques:
  - o Ablation techniques aim to destroy the uterine lining or fibroid tissue to alleviate symptoms such as heavy menstrual bleeding or pelvic pain. These approaches are typically minimally invasive and best suited for women who do not plan to have children in the future.

- o Uterine Artery Embolization (UAE):
  - o This procedure cuts off the blood supply to fibroids, causing them to shrink over time. It is effective for women who wish to avoid surgery but is not suitable for those seeking to preserve fertility.

- o Magnetic Resonance-Guided Focused Ultrasound (MRgFUS):

- o A non-invasive treatment that uses ultrasound waves to heat and destroy fibroid tissue.

3. Surgical Options

- Myomectomy:

    - o A surgical procedure to remove fibroids while preserving the uterus, making it a good option for women desiring future pregnancies. Myomectomy can be performed via open surgery, laparoscopy, or hysteroscopy, depending on the fibroid's size and location.

- Hysterectomy:

    - o The definitive solution for fibroids, involving the removal of the uterus. It is typically reserved for women who have completed their family or have severe symptoms unresponsive to other treatments. This should really only be considered as a very last resort as there are other issues related to removing the uterus.

4. Lifestyle and Natural Remedies

- Dietary Changes:

    - o Consuming a diet rich in fruits, vegetables, and whole grains while limiting grain fed, processed red meat and alcohol may help manage symptoms.

- Stress Management:
  - o Stress may exacerbate hormonal imbalances; therefore, incorporating relaxation techniques such as yoga or meditation can be beneficial.

5. Emerging Treatments

- Advances in robotic surgery and biologics targeting growth pathways in fibroids are promising areas of research.

Factors to Consider When Choosing a Treatment

1. Age and Menopausal Status: Younger women or those approaching menopause may prefer non-invasive treatments since fibroids often shrink naturally post-menopause.

2. Desire for Fertility: Treatments like myomectomy are preferred for women who wish to conceive.

3. Symptom Severity: Women with disabling symptoms may require more definitive solutions like surgery.

4. Health Risks and Comorbidities: Certain treatments may not be safe for women with other medical conditions.

How to Test for Hormonal Imbalances

Understanding and testing for hormonal imbalances is key to diagnosing and managing the conditions mentioned above. Various tests are available, some are to measure the hormones and others are to assess the symptoms visually:

1. **Blood Tests:**

    - **What It Measures:** Blood tests are the most common method for measuring hormone levels such as FSH, LH, oestrogen, progesterone, testosterone, and thyroid hormones.

    - **When It's Used:** In men, the tests can be done any day in the morning. In women, blood tests are typically done on specific days of the menstrual cycle to assess hormone levels accurately. Generally done on day 4 to assess fertility and day 21 to assess oestrogen dominance.

2. **Saliva Testing:**

    - **What It Measures:** Saliva tests measure free, bioavailable hormones, including cortisol, oestrogen, progesterone, and testosterone.

    - **When It's Used:** Saliva tests are often used to assess hormonal fluctuations throughout the day or menstrual cycle, particularly for conditions like PMS, PMDD, and adrenal fatigue.

3. **Dried Urine Testing:**

- **What It Measures:** The dried urine test measures hormone metabolites in urine, providing a comprehensive picture of hormone production, metabolism, and excretion.

- **When It's Used:** This test is useful for diagnosing conditions with complex hormonal imbalances, such as adrenal dysfunction or issues with oestrogen metabolism.

Non-hormone related tests:

4. **Ultrasound and Imaging Tests:**

- **What It Measures:** Pelvic ultrasounds can visualise the ovaries and uterus, helping to diagnose conditions like PCOS and endometriosis.

- **When It's Used:** Ultrasounds are used when physical symptoms suggest a structural or cystic abnormality.

5. **Laparoscopy:**

- **What It Measures:** Laparoscopy is a surgical procedure used to diagnose and sometimes treat endometriosis. It allows direct visualisation of the pelvic organs.

- **When It's Used:** This is typically used when other tests suggest endometriosis or when fertility issues are unexplained.

Causes of Hormonal Imbalances

Hormonal imbalances can result from a variety of factors:

1. **Genetics:** Family history can influence conditions like PCOS, endometriosis, and the timing of menopause. Some genetic mutations in the detox genes can contribute to symptoms.

2. **Stress:** Chronic stress can lead to excess cortisol or adrenal fatigue, disrupting cortisol levels and overall hormonal balance.

3. **Diet and Lifestyle:** Poor diet, lack of exercise, and exposure to environmental toxins can all contribute to hormonal imbalances.

4. **Underlying Health Conditions:** Conditions like thyroid disorders, insulin resistance, and autoimmune diseases can affect hormone production and regulation.

Lifestyle and Nutritional Interventions for Hormonal Health

Supporting hormonal health during the fertile years involves a holistic approach, including lifestyle changes and targeted nutrition.

1. Balanced Diet:

- **Whole Foods:** Focus on a diet rich in whole, unprocessed foods that provide essential nutrients for hormone production and regulation.

- **Anti-inflammatory Foods:** Incorporate foods like leafy greens, berries, fatty fish, and nuts to reduce inflammation.

- **Blood Sugar Balance:** Eat regular meals with a balance of protein, healthy fats, and fibre to maintain stable blood sugar levels.

2. Regular Exercise:

- **Moderate Exercise:** Engage in regular physical activity, such as walking, swimming, or yoga, to support hormonal balance and reduce stress.

- **Strength Training:** Incorporate strength training to build muscle mass and support metabolic health.

3. Stress Management:

- **Mindfulness Practices:** Techniques like meditation, deep breathing, and progressive muscle relaxation can help manage stress and reduce its impact on hormones.

- **Adequate Sleep:** Prioritize sleep by maintaining a consistent sleep schedule and creating a restful sleep environment.

4. Supplements:

- **Vitamin D:** Supports immune function and hormone production. Aim for 1,000 to 2,000 IU daily, or more if levels are low.

- **Magnesium:** Helps with relaxation, stress management, and PMS symptoms. A dose of 200-400 mg daily is typically recommended.

- **Omega-3 Fatty Acids:** Found in fish oil, these support inflammation reduction and hormone balance. Aim for 1,000 to 2,000 mg daily.

- **B Vitamins:** Essential for energy production and hormone metabolism, particularly B6 for PMS relief.

The power of the vaginal microbiome through the life stages:

The vaginal pH and microbiome undergo significant changes throughout a woman's life, influenced by hormonal fluctuations, age, and overall health. These changes can affect vaginal health and predispose to certain conditions when the balance is disrupted. Here's an overview of how vaginal pH and the microbiome change through life stages and how to maintain balance, especially during perimenopause.

1. Childhood (Pre-puberty)

- **Vaginal pH**: Neutral to slightly acidic (around 7).
- **Microbiome**: The vaginal microbiome in young girls is less diverse, often dominated by skin and intestinal bacteria, such as *Staphylococcus* and *Streptococcus* species.
- **Risks**: The higher pH makes the vagina more susceptible to infections, such as vulvovaginitis.

2. Reproductive Years (Puberty to Pre-Menopause)

- **Vaginal pH**: Becomes more acidic, typically around 3.5 to 4.5, due to increased oestrogen levels.
- **Microbiome**: Dominated by *Lactobacillus* species, which produce lactic acid, maintaining a low pH and protecting against pathogens.

- **Risks**: Disruptions in this balance can lead to conditions like bacterial vaginosis (BV), yeast infections, and sexually transmitted infections (STIs).

3. Perimenopause

- **Vaginal pH**: pH begins to rise (towards neutrality) as oestrogen levels fluctuate and eventually decrease.

- **Microbiome**: A decline in *Lactobacillus* species and a potential increase in anaerobic bacteria.

- **Risks**: Higher risk of bacterial vaginosis, atrophic vaginitis (thinning and inflammation of vaginal walls), and increased susceptibility to infections due to a less acidic environment.

4. Menopause and Post-Menopause

- **Vaginal pH**: Often becomes more neutral, around 6 to 7, due to low oestrogen levels.

- **Microbiome**: Further reduction in *Lactobacillus* with an increase in diversity of other bacteria, including pathogens.

- **Risks**: Increased risk of urogenital infections, dryness, irritation, and conditions like atrophic vaginitis and urinary tract infections (UTIs).

Conditions Linked to Disrupted Vaginal Microbiome

- **Bacterial Vaginosis (BV)**: Imbalance with an overgrowth of anaerobic bacteria and reduced *Lactobacillus*, leading to a higher pH.

- **Yeast Infections**: Overgrowth of *Candida* species, often triggered by changes in pH, antibiotic use, or hormonal fluctuations.

- **Atrophic Vaginitis**: Inflammation and thinning of the vaginal walls due to decreased oestrogen, common during and after menopause.

- **Urinary Tract Infections (UTIs)**: Disrupted microbiome and pH can increase susceptibility to UTIs, especially during menopause.

Maintaining Vaginal Health Through Perimenopause

1. **Hormonal Support**:

   - **Topical Oestrogen**: Localised oestrogen therapy can help maintain the health of the vaginal lining, keeping it thick and acidic.

   - **Hormone Replacement Therapy (HRT)**: Systemic HRT may be considered to manage broader menopausal symptoms, which can indirectly benefit vaginal health.

2. **Probiotics**:

- Oral or vaginal probiotics containing *Lactobacillus* species can help restore and maintain a healthy vaginal microbiome. The best and most well researched probiotics for vaginal health are Lactobacillus crispatus LCR01 (DSM 24619), Lactobacillus fermentum LF10 (DSM 19187) and Lactobacillus acidophilus LA02 (DSM 21712).

3. **Hydration and Lubrication**:

   o **Vaginal Moisturisers**: Regular use can help combat dryness and maintain the vaginal environment.

   o **Water-Based Lubricants**: Especially during sexual activity to reduce friction and prevent microtraumas.

4. **Lifestyle and Diet**:

   o **Balanced Diet**: Diets rich in prebiotics (fibre), probiotics (yogurt, fermented foods), and phytoestrogens (soy) can support the microbiome.

   o **Regular Exercise**: Promotes overall circulation and hormonal balance.

   o **Avoiding Irritants**: Such as douches, scented products, and harsh soaps that can disrupt pH and microbiome balance.

5. **Regular Check-ups**:

- o Regular gynaecological visits can help monitor vaginal health and address any changes or symptoms early.

- o **Vaginal microbiome** tests are now readily available, and you can ask your healthcare provider to order one for you if you suspect an imbalance that can be treated with probiotics.

Maintaining vaginal health during perimenopause and beyond involves proactive management of hormonal changes, supporting the microbiome, and addressing symptoms as they arise. This approach can help reduce the risk of infections and maintain comfort and well-being.

Conclusion:

The fertile years are a time of both opportunity and challenge when it comes to hormonal health. By understanding the conditions that can arise, recognising the importance of appropriate testing, and embracing lifestyle and nutritional interventions, women can take proactive steps to support their well-being during this pivotal phase of life.

Chapter 12

Male Hormones in the Fertile Years: Understanding Conditions, Tests, and Nutritional Support

Introduction: The Role of Hormones in Men's Health

The fertile years, typically from the late teens through the early forties, are a crucial period for men's health, particularly concerning hormonal balance. During these years, male hormones, primarily testosterone, play a vital role in physical development, sexual health, mood, energy levels, and overall well-being. Understanding how these hormones function, the conditions that can arise from imbalances, how to test for these imbalances, and the lifestyle and nutritional strategies to support optimal hormone health is essential for maintaining vitality during these years.

This chapter explores common hormonal conditions in men during the fertile years, including fertility issues, low testosterone and other endocrine disorders. We will discuss the tests available for diagnosing these conditions, the main causes, and the lifestyle and nutritional interventions that can help support hormonal balance and improve health outcomes.

Key Hormonal Conditions During the Fertile Years

1. Low Testosterone (Hypogonadism):

- **Overview:** Testosterone is the primary male sex hormone, essential for sexual development, muscle growth, bone density, and overall energy levels. Hypogonadism occurs when the body produces insufficient testosterone.

- **Symptoms:** Symptoms of low testosterone include reduced libido, erectile dysfunction, fatigue, depression, loss of muscle mass, increased body fat, and decreased bone density.

- **Causes:** Low testosterone can result from a variety of factors, including aging, obesity, chronic stress, certain medications, and underlying medical conditions such as diabetes or pituitary disorders.

- **Testing:** Blood tests measuring total and free testosterone levels, along with luteinizing hormone (LH) and follicle-stimulating hormone (FSH) levels, are typically used to diagnose hypogonadism.

- **Lifestyle Interventions:** Regular exercise, particularly strength training, maintaining a healthy weight, and managing stress can help boost testosterone levels naturally.

o **Nutritional Support:** A diet rich in zinc, magnesium, vitamin D, and healthy fats (such as omega-3 fatty acids) supports testosterone production. Avoiding excessive alcohol, sugar, and processed foods is also beneficial.

2. **Fertility Challenges:**

   o **Overview:** Male fertility is primarily influenced by the quantity and quality of sperm, which is regulated by testosterone and other hormones like FSH and LH.

   o **Symptoms:** Difficulty conceiving, low sperm count, poor sperm motility, and erectile dysfunction are common indicators of fertility issues.

   o **Causes:** Causes can include hormonal imbalances, genetic factors, lifestyle choices (such as smoking and excessive alcohol consumption), environmental toxins, and conditions like varicocele or infections.

   o **Testing:** Semen analysis is the primary test for evaluating male fertility, assessing sperm count, motility, and morphology. Hormone testing may also be conducted to assess testosterone, FSH, and LH levels.

   o **Lifestyle Interventions:** Avoiding smoking, limiting alcohol intake, maintaining a healthy weight, and reducing stress can significantly improve fertility. Regular physical activity is also crucial.

- ○ **Nutritional Support:** Antioxidants like vitamin C and E, zinc, selenium, and omega-3 fatty acids are important for sperm health. Supplements such as CoQ10 and L-carnitine may also enhance sperm quality.

3. **Andropause (Male Menopause):**
   - ○ **Overview:** Andropause refers to the gradual decline in testosterone levels that can occur as men age, typically starting in their late thirties or early forties. While not as abrupt as female menopause, andropause can still lead to significant changes.

   - ○ **Symptoms:** Symptoms include reduced libido, fatigue, mood swings, irritability, loss of muscle mass, increased body fat, and reduced cognitive function.

   - ○ **Causes:** Andropause is primarily due to aging and the natural decline in testosterone production. Lifestyle factors such as poor diet, lack of exercise, and chronic stress can exacerbate the symptoms.

   - ○ **Testing:** Blood tests to measure testosterone levels, along with other relevant hormones, such as SHBG (sex hormone-binding globulin), are used to diagnose andropause.

- o **Lifestyle Interventions:** Regular physical activity, particularly strength training, stress management, and adequate sleep are key to managing the symptoms of andropause.

- o **Nutritional Support:** A diet rich in good quality proteins, healthy fats, and micronutrients like vitamin D, zinc, and magnesium can help support testosterone levels. Reducing intake of refined sugars and processed foods is also important.

4. **Metabolic Syndrome:**

- o **Overview:** Metabolic syndrome is a cluster of conditions, including high blood pressure, high blood sugar, excess body fat around the waist, and abnormal cholesterol levels. It is closely linked to low testosterone levels and can increase the risk of cardiovascular disease and diabetes.

- o **Symptoms:** Symptoms include increased waist circumference, high fasting blood sugar, high blood pressure, and abnormal cholesterol levels.

- o **Causes:** Metabolic syndrome is often the result of insulin resistance, poor diet, lack of physical activity, and genetic factors. Low testosterone is both a contributing factor and a consequence of metabolic syndrome.

- ○ **Testing:** Blood tests to assess fasting glucose, lipid profiles, and testosterone levels are used to diagnose metabolic syndrome.

- ○ **Lifestyle Interventions:** Weight loss through diet and exercise is crucial for managing metabolic syndrome. Regular physical activity, particularly cardiovascular and resistance training, helps improve insulin sensitivity and hormone balance.

- ○ **Nutritional Support:** A diet low in refined carbohydrates and high in fibre, healthy fats, and good quality proteins is recommended. Nutrients like chromium, magnesium, and omega-3 fatty acids can help regulate blood sugar levels and improve metabolic health.

How to Test for Hormonal Imbalances

Accurate testing is essential for diagnosing hormonal imbalances and developing an effective treatment plan. Here are the primary tests used for evaluating male hormone levels:

1. **Blood Tests:**

   o **What It Measures:** Blood tests are the standard method for measuring hormone levels, including total and free testosterone, LH, FSH, SHBG, PSA and prolactin.

   o **When It's Used:** Blood tests are usually done in the morning when testosterone levels are highest. They are essential for diagnosing low testosterone, hypogonadism, and assessing fertility-related issues.

2. **Semen Analysis:**

   o **What It Measures:** Semen analysis evaluates sperm count, motility, and morphology, providing critical information about male fertility.

   o **When It's Used:** This test is used when there are concerns about fertility or when a couple is experiencing difficulty conceiving.

3. **Saliva Testing:**

   o **What It Measures:** Saliva tests can measure free testosterone and cortisol levels, providing insight into hormone levels at different times of the day.

o **When It's Used:** Saliva testing is sometimes used for assessing daily hormone fluctuations and adrenal function.

4. **Dried Urine Testing:**

   o **What It Measures:** The dried urine test measures hormone metabolites in urine, offering a comprehensive picture of hormone production, metabolism, and excretion.

   o **When It's Used:** This test is particularly useful for understanding complex hormonal imbalances and adrenal function.

5. **Imaging Tests:**

   o **What It Measures:** Ultrasound or MRI can be used to evaluate the testes and pituitary gland if there are concerns about structural abnormalities affecting hormone production.

   o **When It's Used:** Imaging is used when blood tests and symptoms suggest an underlying physical issue, such as a pituitary tumour or varicocele.

Causes of Hormonal Imbalances

Hormonal imbalances in men during the fertile years can result from a variety of factors:

1. **Aging:** Testosterone levels naturally decline with age, leading to symptoms associated with andropause.

2. **Lifestyle Factors:** Poor diet, lack of exercise, chronic stress, and exposure to environmental toxins can all contribute to hormonal imbalances.

3. **Medical Conditions:** Conditions such as diabetes, obesity, metabolic syndrome, and chronic illnesses can disrupt hormone production and regulation.

4. **Medications:** Certain medications, such as corticosteroids, opioids, and anabolic steroids, can negatively impact testosterone levels.

5. **Genetics:** Genetic factors may predispose some men to conditions like hypogonadism or low testosterone.

Lifestyle and Nutritional Interventions for Hormonal Health

Supporting hormonal health during the fertile years involves making conscious lifestyle choices and ensuring proper nutrition:

1. Balanced Diet:

- **Whole Foods:** A diet rich in whole, unprocessed foods provides the essential nutrients needed for hormone production and regulation.

- **Healthy Fats:** Incorporate sources of healthy fats, such as avocados, nuts, seeds, and fatty fish, which are crucial for testosterone production.

- **Zinc and Magnesium:** Foods rich in zinc (like lean meats, shellfish, and legumes) and magnesium (such as leafy greens, nuts, and seeds) support testosterone levels and overall hormone health.

- **Antioxidants:** Vitamins C and E, along with selenium and CoQ10, can protect sperm and testosterone production from oxidative stress.

2. Regular Exercise:

- **Strength Training:** Resistance exercises, such as weightlifting, can significantly boost testosterone levels and improve muscle mass.

- **Cardiovascular Activity:** Regular aerobic exercise supports cardiovascular health and helps maintain a healthy weight, which is crucial for hormone balance.

- **Active Recovery:** Incorporating stretching, yoga, or light activities helps reduce stress and supports overall well-being.

3. Stress Management:

- **Mindfulness Practices:** Meditation, deep breathing exercises, and mindfulness practices can help reduce stress, which negatively impacts testosterone levels.

- **Adequate Sleep:** Prioritize sleep by maintaining a consistent sleep schedule, which is essential for hormone production and recovery.

- **Balanced Work-Life:** Ensuring a healthy work-life balance can prevent chronic stress, a significant contributor to hormonal imbalances.

4. Avoiding Toxins:

- **Reduce Exposure:** Limit exposure to endocrine-disrupting chemicals found in plastics, pesticides, and personal care products.

- **Detoxification:** Supporting liver function with foods like cruciferous vegetables, garlic, and green tea can help detoxify harmful substances that impact hormone health.

Conclusion:

Men's fertile years are a time when maintaining hormonal balance is crucial for overall health, fertility, and vitality. Understanding the potential challenges, recognising the signs of hormonal imbalances, and implementing effective testing and interventions can help men navigate this period with greater ease.

By adopting a balanced lifestyle and focusing on proper nutrition, men can support their hormonal health and ensure they remain strong, vital, and healthy during these years and beyond.

Chapter 13

Understanding Contraception: Options, Pros and Cons, and Supporting Your Body with Nutrition and Lifestyle

Introduction: The Importance of Contraception

Contraception is a crucial aspect of reproductive health, allowing individuals to make informed decisions about if and when they want to conceive, but also have a conversation about sexual health in general and the prevention of sexually transmitted diseases. With a wide range of contraceptive options available today, it's important to understand the different methods, their effectiveness, potential side effects, and how they align with your lifestyle and health goals.

In this chapter, we will explore the various forms of contraception, both hormonal and non-hormonal, examining their pros and cons. Additionally, we'll discuss how nutrition and lifestyle choices can support your body while using contraception, helping to mitigate any potential negative effects.

Let's start with options for Men!

Other than condoms, you're probably wondering what I'm talking about! There are 2 worth discussing, one is surgical and permanent and the other is temporary. The temporary one is called ADAM™ and was launched in 2024. How it works, is the man gets a hydrogel injected (with anesthetic) into the vas deferens (the tube that carries the sperm to the penis from the scrotum), the same tube that can be cut in a vasectomy (the other, but more permanent form of male contraception). This then blocks the sperm without affecting sensation or ejaculation! The blocked sperm simply degrade and get reabsorbed into the body.

At the end of its lifespan, the hydrogel liquefies, removing the barrier and sperm is then free to flow again.

It has so many more benefits that anything offered to women and will hopefully become the gold standard for contraception in the future as it is non-hormonal, quick and easy!

And now for the ladies:

There are a number of ways you can prevent pregnancy, they include the use of hormones and of course, there are non-hormonal methods. The pros and cons of each are discussed below.

Hormonal Contraception: How It Works and What to Consider

Hormonal contraception methods work by altering the body's natural hormone levels to prevent ovulation, thicken cervical mucus, or alter the uterine lining, making it less hospitable for a fertilised egg.

1. Oral Contraceptives (The Pill):

- **Types:** Combination pills (containing oestrogen and progestin) and progestin-only pills (also known as the mini-pill).

- **How It Works:** The combination pill prevents ovulation, thickens cervical mucus, and thins the uterine lining. The mini-pill mainly works by thickening cervical mucus and sometimes suppressing ovulation.

- **Pros:**
  - High effectiveness when taken consistently.
  - Can regulate menstrual cycles and reduce symptoms of PMS.
  - May reduce the risk of ovarian and endometrial cancers.

- **Cons:**
  - ○ Requires daily adherence.
  - ○ Possible side effects include nausea, headaches, mood changes, and an increased risk of blood clots, particularly in smokers or women over 35.
  - ○ May deplete certain nutrients like B vitamins, magnesium, and zinc.
  - ○ Reduced effectiveness with certain medications.
  - ○ May increase the risk of certain oestrogenic cancers.

2. Hormonal Intrauterine Device (IUD):

- **Types:** IUDs like Mirena, Skyla, Liletta, and Kyleena release progestin, a synthetic form of progesterone made in a lab.
- **How It Works:** The progestin thickens cervical mucus, inhibits sperm movement, and thins the uterine lining, preventing fertilisation and implantation.
- **Pros:**
  - ○ Long-term protection (3-7 years, depending on the type).
  - ○ Low maintenance: once inserted, no daily action is required.

- o Can reduce menstrual bleeding and cramps.

- **Cons:**

  - o Potential side effects include irregular bleeding, spotting, or discomfort during insertion.

  - o Rare complications include perforation of the uterus or expulsion of the IUD.

  - o Serious symptoms of Mirena IUD removal are prolonged or severe pain in the uterus or abdomen, fever, excessive bleeding, anxiety, depression, and mood swings.

3. The Contraceptive Patch:

- **How It Works:** A combination of oestrogen and progestin delivered through the skin, preventing ovulation.

- **Pros:**

  - o Weekly application; no daily pill required.

  - o Can regulate menstrual cycles.

- **Cons:**

  - o Possible skin irritation at the application site.

  - o May increase the risk of blood clots, particularly in women who smoke or are over 35.

  - o Visible on the skin, which some may find inconvenient.

4. The Vaginal Ring (NuvaRing):

- **How It Works**: A flexible ring inserted into the vagina that releases oestrogen and progestin to prevent ovulation.

- **Pros:**
  - Monthly application (left in place for three weeks).
  - May improve menstrual symptoms and reduce acne.

- **Cons:**
  - Potential for vaginal irritation or discharge.
  - Must be comfortable with self-insertion and removal.
  - Similar risks as other combination hormonal contraceptives.

5. The Contraceptive Injection (Depo-Provera):

- **How It Works:** An injection of progestin administered every three months, preventing ovulation and thickening cervical mucus.

- **Pros:**
  - Effective and requires only four injections per year.
  - May reduce the risk of endometrial cancer and improve symptoms of endometriosis.

- **Cons:**
  - ○ Potential for significant weight gain, mood changes, and decreased bone density with long-term use.
  - ○ Can delay the return to fertility after stopping the injections.

6. The Contraceptive Implant (Nexplanon):

- **How It Works:** A small rod inserted under the skin of the upper arm, releasing progestin to prevent ovulation and thicken cervical mucus.

- **Pros:**
  - ○ Long-term protection (up to 3 years).
  - ○ Highly effective and low maintenance.

- **Cons:**
  - ○ Irregular bleeding is common, especially in the first year.
  - ○ Requires a minor surgical procedure for insertion and removal.
  - ○ Possible side effects include weight gain, acne, and mood changes.

Non-Hormonal Contraception: Alternatives for Those Seeking Hormone-Free Options

For individuals who prefer not to use hormones, there are several effective non-hormonal contraceptive methods available.

1. Copper Intrauterine Device (IUD):

- **How It Works:** The copper IUD (Paragard) releases copper ions, which are toxic to sperm, preventing fertilisation.

- **Pros:**
  - Long-term protection (up to 10 years).
  - Hormone-free and doesn't affect the menstrual cycle.
  - Can be used as emergency contraception if inserted within five days of unprotected sex.

- **Cons:**
  - May cause heavier, longer, and more painful periods, particularly in the first few months.
  - Insertion can be uncomfortable, and there is a small risk of perforation or expulsion.

- o If you are already copper toxic it can increase any associated symptoms such as nausea and moodiness.

2. Barrier Methods:

- **Types:** Condoms (male and female), diaphragms, and cervical caps.

- **How They Work:** These methods physically block sperm from reaching the egg. Condoms also protect against sexually transmitted infections (STIs).

- **Pros:**
  - o No hormones or long-term commitment.
  - o Condoms are readily available and inexpensive.
  - o Some methods can be used only when needed, without affecting fertility.

- **Cons:**
  - o Less effective than hormonal methods when used inconsistently or incorrectly.
  - o Can interrupt spontaneity during sexual activity.
  - o Some people may be allergic to latex or find barrier methods uncomfortable.

3. Fertility Awareness Methods (FAMs):

- **How They Work:** FAMs involve tracking the menstrual cycle to determine fertile days, during which other forms of contraception or abstinence are practiced.

- **Pros:**
  - No hormones or devices.
  - Empowers individuals to understand their reproductive cycles.

- **Cons:**
  - Requires meticulous tracking and discipline. There are a number of App's available that can help track when you are fertile but they need to be used consistently to be accurate.
  - Less effective if not followed consistently.
  - Does not protect against STIs.

4. Permanent Methods:

- **Types:** Tubal ligation for women and vasectomy for men.

- **How They Work:** Surgical procedures that permanently prevent the sperm from reaching the egg. Tubal ligation blocks the fallopian tubes, while vasectomy cuts and seals the vas deferens.

- **Pros:**
  - Permanent solution with very high effectiveness.
  - No ongoing maintenance required.

- **Cons:**
  - Irreversible; should be considered only by those certain they do not want future pregnancies.
  - Surgical risks, including complications from anaesthesia and infection.

Supporting Your Body with Nutrition and Lifestyle

While contraception is essential for family planning and sexual health, it can have various side effects that impact overall well-being. Whatever decision you make regarding contraception, nutrition and lifestyle choices can play a significant role in mitigating potential negative effects from the hormonal and copper devices while supporting your reproductive health.

1. Nutritional Support:

- **B Vitamins:** Hormonal contraceptives, particularly oral contraceptives, can deplete B vitamins (such as B6, B12, and folate). Incorporating foods rich in B vitamins (like leafy greens, whole grains, eggs, and fortified cereals) or taking a B-complex supplement can help.

- **Magnesium:** Contraceptive use can also deplete magnesium, which is essential for mood regulation, sleep, and muscle function. Foods like nuts, seeds, whole grains, and dark chocolate are good sources of magnesium.

- **Zinc:** Hormonal contraceptives may lower zinc levels, which are crucial for immune function and hormone balance. Include zinc-rich foods like oysters, red meat, beans, and nuts in your diet.

- **Antioxidants:** To counteract the oxidative stress that can be induced by some contraceptive methods, a diet rich in antioxidants is beneficial. This includes plenty of fruits and vegetables, especially those high in vitamins C and E, like berries, citrus fruits, nuts, and seeds.

- **Healthy Fats:** Omega-3 fatty acids, found in fatty fish, flaxseeds, and walnuts, support hormone production and reduce inflammation. These are particularly important for those using hormonal contraception, which can sometimes lead to inflammatory conditions.

- **Fibre:** Adequate fibre intake supports detoxification processes, particularly in the liver, where hormones are metabolised. Whole grains, legumes, fruits, and vegetables are excellent sources of fibre.

2. Lifestyle Habits:

- **Exercise:** Regular physical activity supports overall hormonal balance, improves mood, and helps maintain a healthy weight, which is important for reproductive health. Incorporating a mix of cardiovascular exercise, strength training, and flexibility exercises like yoga can be particularly beneficial.

- **Stress** Management: High stress levels can exacerbate side effects of contraceptives, particularly mood-related issues. Mindfulness practices, deep breathing, and activities that promote relaxation, such as meditation and yoga, can help manage stress.

- **Sleep:** Adequate sleep is essential for hormonal regulation and overall health. Aim for 7-9 hours of quality sleep per night and establish a regular sleep routine to support your body while using contraception.

- **Hydration:** Staying well-hydrated helps the body detoxify and can alleviate some side effects of hormonal contraceptives, such as bloating and headaches. Aim for at least 8 glasses of water per day.

- **Regular Check-Ups:** Regular visits to your healthcare provider can help monitor any side effects or complications from contraceptive use. They can **also**

provide guidance on managing side effects through diet, lifestyle changes, or adjustments in contraceptive methods.

Conclusion:

Choosing the right contraceptive method is a personal decision that depends on various factors, including health, lifestyle, and family planning goals. By understanding the options available, the pros and cons of each, and how to support your body through nutrition and lifestyle, you can make informed choices that align with your needs.

It's important to regularly review your contraceptive choices with your healthcare provider, especially if your health status or family planning goals change. Remember, the best contraceptive method is one that you feel comfortable with, that suits your lifestyle, and that you can use consistently and correctly.

Chapter 14

Preparing for Pregnancy: Optimising Health for a Healthy Baby

Introduction: The Importance of Preparation

Preparing for pregnancy is a crucial time that involves more than just deciding to have a baby. It's about creating the healthiest possible environment for both conception and foetal development. The months leading up to pregnancy, often referred to as the preconception period, provide a unique opportunity to optimise health, address any existing issues, and lay the foundation for a healthy pregnancy and baby.

This chapter will explore the key aspects of future parents preparing for pregnancy, including understanding folliculogenesis (the development of ovarian follicles) in women, the importance of removing toxins like heavy metals in both parents, and the role of nutrition and lifestyle habits in ensuring the best possible outcomes for both parents and thechild.

Future fathers should follow the advice in chapter 8 to ensure healthy sperm.

Understanding Folliculogenesis

1. **What is Folliculogenesis?**

   o **Overview:** Folliculogenesis is the process by which ovarian follicles (immature eggs) mature and prepare an egg for ovulation. It begins during a woman's foetal development (when she is in her mom's uterus!), with a finite number of primordial follicles formed in the ovaries, which will later mature into eggs during a woman's reproductive years. It is so important to respect that fact that a pregnant women who is having a baby girl, has 2 future generations inside her! She has her baby and her baby's eggs!

   o **Phases:** Folliculogenesis occurs in several phases:

      ▪ **Primordial Follicles:** These are the most immature follicles present in the ovaries from birth, yes, they are in the baby girl from birth. From puberty, a group of these follicules start the marathon, where one (not all, the rest self-destruct) will end up winning the race of becoming a healthy egg!

      ▪ **Primary Follicles:** These follicles begin to develop at the onset of puberty, growing slightly larger and starting to produce the hormone oestrogen. One of these will eventually become the healthy egg.

- **Secondary Follicles:** These follicles continue to grow, and their cells multiply, further increasing oestrogen production. At this point, they need very good nutrient information from the future mom to ensure the egg is healthy.

- **Antral Follicles:** These follicles form a fluid-filled cavity (antrum) and continue to mature. One of these follicles will become dominant and is selected for ovulation, she is the winner and is hopefully a healthy egg.

- **Graafian Follicle:** The fully matured follicle, the winner of the race, is now ready for ovulation. During ovulation, the Graafian follicle releases the healthy egg, which then travels down the fallopian tube for potential fertilisation.

2. Why is Folliculogenesis Important for Pregnancy?

- **Egg Quality:** The quality of the egg released during ovulation is directly related to the health of the follicles. Healthy folliculogenesis ensures that the egg is of high quality, which is crucial for successful fertilisation, embryo development, and a healthy pregnancy.

- o **Hormonal Balance:** Proper folliculogenesis is essential for maintaining hormonal balance, particularly the production of oestrogen and progesterone, which are vital for preparing the uterine lining for implantation and supporting early pregnancy.

- o **Timing:** The timing of folliculogenesis aligns with the menstrual cycle, ensuring that ovulation occurs at the optimal time for conception.

The Role of Detoxification:

Removing Toxins for a Healthy Pregnancy

1. **Understanding Environmental Toxins:**

- o **Heavy Metals:** Exposure to heavy metals such as lead, mercury, and cadmium can negatively impact fertility, egg quality, and foetal development. These metals can accumulate in the body over time and disrupt hormonal balance, damage DNA, and interfere with the body's natural detoxification processes.

- o **Endocrine Disruptors:** Chemicals found in plastics (like BPA), pesticides, and certain personal care products can mimic or interfere with the body's natural hormones, potentially leading to fertility issues and complications during pregnancy.

o **Other Toxins:** Pollutants, chemicals in cleaning products, and even certain foods can introduce toxins into the body that may affect reproductive health and foetal development.

2. **Why Detoxification Matters:**

o **Reducing Toxic Load:** Detoxification helps reduce the body's toxic load, improving overall health and creating a safer environment for conception and pregnancy.

o **Enhancing Egg Quality:** By reducing the levels of toxins in the body, the chances of healthy folliculogenesis and egg development are increased, which can improve the likelihood of a healthy pregnancy.

o **Protecting Foetal Development:** Early foetal development is highly sensitive to environmental toxins. By detoxifying before pregnancy, you can reduce the risk of complications and developmental issues in the baby.

3. **How to Detoxify Safely:**

   o **Dietary Changes:** Incorporating organic foods, particularly fruits and vegetables, can help reduce exposure to pesticides and other harmful chemicals. Foods rich in antioxidants (like berries, leafy greens, and nuts) support the body's natural detoxification processes.

   o **Hydration:** Drinking plenty of filtered water helps flush toxins from the body. Incorporating herbal teas with detoxifying properties (such as dandelion root or milk thistle) can further support liver function.

   o **Sweating:** Regular exercise and activities like sauna sessions promote sweating, which is a natural way for the body to eliminate toxins.

   o **Avoiding Toxins:** Reduce exposure to known toxins by using natural or organic cleaning and personal care products, avoiding plastics, and choosing low-mercury fish.

   o **Supplements:** Supplements like glutathione, NAC (N-acetylcysteine), and activated charcoal can support detoxification. However, it's important to consult with a healthcare provider before starting any detox regimen.

Nutrition: Fuelling Fertility and Supporting Pregnancy

1. **Key Nutrients for Preconception:**

   o **Folate (Vitamin B9):** Essential for DNA synthesis and repair, folate is crucial for preventing neural tube defects in the developing foetus. Women planning to conceive should take 400-800 mcg of folate daily, ideally in the form of methylated folate for better absorption.

   o **Iron:** Iron supports the production of haemoglobin, which is necessary for oxygen transport in the blood. Adequate iron levels are important for preventing anaemia during pregnancy. Include iron-rich foods like lean meats, beans, and fortified cereals in your diet.

   o **Calcium and Vitamin D:** These nutrients are critical for bone health, both for the mother and the developing baby. Calcium-rich foods include dairy products, leafy greens, and fortified plant-based milks. Vitamin D can be obtained from sun exposure and foods like fatty fish, eggs, and fortified products.

   o **Omega-3 Fatty Acids:** Omega-3s, particularly DHA, are vital for brain development in the foetus. Include sources like fatty fish (such as salmon), flaxseeds, chia seeds, and walnuts in your diet.

- ○ **Zinc:** Zinc supports hormone production, immune function, and cell division, all of which are important for fertility and pregnancy. Foods high in zinc include oysters, red meat, poultry, and seeds.

2. **The Importance of a Balanced Diet:**

- ○ **Whole Foods:** A diet rich in whole, unprocessed foods provides the essential vitamins, minerals, and antioxidants needed for reproductive health and a healthy pregnancy.

- ○ **Healthy Fats:** Incorporate healthy fats, such as avocados, nuts, seeds, and olive oil, to support hormone production and overall health.

- ○ **Low Glycaemic Index Foods:** Choosing low-glycaemic index foods, such as proteins, whole grains, legumes, and non-starchy vegetables, helps regulate blood sugar levels and supports metabolic health, which is important for fertility.

3. **Supplements for Preconception:**

- ○ **Prenatal Vitamins:** A high-quality prenatal vitamin provides essential nutrients like folate, zinc, iron, calcium, choline and DHA (for brain health), ensuring that the mother has adequate levels before and during pregnancy. The only vitamin to be cautious of is Vitamin A.

o Getting the right amount of vitamin A while pregnant is a bit of a balancing act. Too much can harm your developing baby and lead to birth defects, while too little carries certain risks to you and your baby's development. A healthy intake will ensure that your baby gets the nutritional support they need for normal growth and development.

o Pregnant women need a little more vitamin A in pregnancy than they usually would. The daily RNI of vitamin A for pregnant women is 700 micrograms, which is 100 micrograms more than for the average female adult. To put this into context, half a cup of raw carrots contains 459 micrograms of vitamin A, and half a cup of broccoli contains 60 micrograms of vitamin A.

o There's no reason why you can't get all the vitamin A you need from the foods you eat in your diet, although you don't need a supply of it every day. This is because vitamin A is a fat-soluble vitamin that your body can build up stores of in your liver. As such, any vitamin A your body doesn't use straight away is stored away to be used in the future. If you're concerned at all about your Vitamin A intake, please get the advice of a qualified nutritional therapist.

o **Probiotics:** A healthy gut microbiome is important for overall health and can influence pregnancy outcomes. Probiotic supplements or fermented foods like yogurt, kefir, and sauerkraut can support gut health.

o **Antioxidants:** Antioxidant supplements, such as vitamins C and E, CoQ10, and selenium, can help protect eggs and sperm from oxidative stress, improving fertility outcomes.

Lifestyle Habits for a Healthy Pregnancy

1. **Regular Exercise:**

o **Benefits:** Regular physical activity supports cardiovascular health, helps maintain a healthy weight, and reduces stress, all of which are important for fertility and pregnancy.

o **Types of Exercise:** Aim for a mix of cardiovascular exercise (like walking, swimming, or cycling) and strength training. Yoga and Pilates can also be beneficial for improving flexibility, reducing stress, and preparing the body for pregnancy.

2. **Stress Management:**

   o **Impact of Stress:** Chronic stress can disrupt hormonal balance, impair ovulation, and negatively affect fertility. It's important to develop strategies for managing stress during the preconception period.

   o **Stress Reduction Techniques:** Meditation, deep breathing exercises, mindfulness practices, and activities like yoga or tai chi can help reduce stress levels. Ensuring adequate sleep and maintaining a healthy work-life balance are also crucial.

3. **Avoiding Harmful Substances:**

   o **Smoking:** Smoking is linked to reduced fertility, increased risk of miscarriage, and complications during pregnancy. Quitting smoking is one of the most important steps you can take when preparing for pregnancy.

   o **Alcohol:** Alcohol consumption can negatively impact fertility and increase the risk of birth defects. It's advisable to limit or avoid alcohol when trying to conceive.

- o **Caffeine:** While moderate caffeine consumption is generally considered safe, excessive caffeine can affect fertility and increase the risk of miscarriage. Aim to limit intake to 200 mg per day (about one 12-ounce cup of coffee).

4. **Environmental Considerations:**

   - o **Reducing Exposure to Endocrine Disruptors:** Choose products that are free from harmful chemicals, such as BPA, phthalates, and parabens, which can interfere with hormone balance.

   - o **Home Environment:** Consider using air purifiers, avoiding synthetic fragrances, and using natural cleaning products to reduce exposure to toxins in your home.

Staying healthy during your Pregnancy

Pregnancy can be a breeze for some women, however, in others, can bring various symptoms such as nausea, fatigue, heartburn, and back pain. While it's always important to consult a healthcare provider before making significant changes, there are several natural tips and lifestyle adjustments that can help alleviate common pregnancy symptoms.

1. Nausea and Morning Sickness

Nausea, especially in the first trimester, is one of the most common symptoms during pregnancy. Here are some natural ways to manage it:

- **Eat Small, Frequent Meals**: Instead of three large meals, try eating smaller meals throughout the day to keep your stomach from becoming too full or too empty.

- **Ginger**: Ginger tea, ginger chews, or ginger supplements (with a doctor's approval) can reduce nausea.

- **Vitamin B6**: This vitamin has been shown to help reduce nausea. Foods like bananas, avocados, and whole grains are rich in B6.

- **Stay Hydrated**: Sip on water throughout the day. If plain water worsens nausea, try flavoured water or herbal teas like peppermint or chamomile.

2. Fatigue

Fatigue is common, especially during the first and third trimesters.

- **Prioritise Rest**: Listen to your body and rest when needed. If possible, take naps during the day.

- **Eat Iron-Rich Foods**: Fatigue can be linked to low iron levels, so include iron-rich foods like spinach, lentils, and lean meats. Pair with vitamin C-rich foods (citrus fruits, bell peppers) to improve iron absorption.

- **Exercise**: Gentle activities like walking, prenatal yoga, or swimming can increase energy levels and reduce fatigue.

- **Stay Hydrated**: Dehydration can worsen fatigue, so ensure you're drinking enough water throughout the day.

3. Heartburn

Heartburn is often caused by hormonal changes that relax the muscles in the oesophagus, as well as the growing uterus putting pressure on the stomach.

- **Eat Smaller Meals**: Smaller, frequent meals can prevent the stomach from becoming overly full, reducing the likelihood of heartburn.

- **Avoid Trigger Foods**: Common triggers include spicy foods, citrus, caffeine, and fatty or fried foods.

- **Sit Up After Eating**: Stay upright for at least 30 minutes after eating to help food digest properly.

- **Elevate Your Head While Sleeping**: Elevating your head and upper body while sleeping can prevent stomach acid from rising.

4. Constipation

Hormonal changes and the pressure of the growing baby on the intestines can lead to constipation.

- **Increase Fibre Intake**: Eat plenty of fibre-rich foods like fruits, vegetables, whole grains, and legumes.

- **Stay Hydrated**: Drink plenty of water to keep things moving through your digestive tract.

- **Prunes or Prune Juice**: Prunes are a natural remedy for constipation and can help stimulate bowel movements.

- **Magnesium citrate**: This form of magnesium is safe and can soften the stool.

- **Exercise**: Gentle exercise like walking or yoga can help promote healthy digestion.

5. Back Pain

As your baby grows, the added weight can strain your back muscles and affect your posture.

- **Maintain Good Posture**: Avoid slouching. Stand and sit with your back straight and shoulders back. Support your lower back with a cushion when sitting.

- **Prenatal Yoga or Stretching**: Gentle stretches and prenatal yoga can relieve back pain by improving flexibility and strength.

- **Use a Maternity Belt**: A supportive belt can help alleviate some of the pressure on your lower back.
- **Sleep on Your Side**: Use a pregnancy pillow or extra cushions to support your belly and back while sleeping.
- **Massage**: Many massage therapists specialise in pregnancy massage, seek one out and treat yourself.

6. Leg Cramps

Leg cramps are common, especially at night, due to the added pressure on blood vessels and nerves.

- **Stretch Your Legs**: Stretching your calf muscles before bed can help prevent cramps.
- **Magnesium**: Ensure you're getting enough magnesium, which can help with muscle relaxation. You can get magnesium from foods like leafy greens, nuts, seeds, and whole grains, or through supplements if suggested by your healthcare provider.
- **Stay Hydrated**: Drink plenty of water throughout the day to prevent dehydration, a common cause of cramps.

7. Swelling

Swelling in the feet, ankles, and hands is common, particularly later in pregnancy.

- **Elevate Your Legs**: When sitting or resting, elevate your legs to improve circulation and reduce swelling.

- **Stay Hydrated**: Drinking more water can help flush out excess fluids and reduce swelling.

- **Wear Comfortable Shoes**: Choose supportive shoes with enough room for your feet to expand.

- **Compression Stockings**: These can help reduce swelling and improve circulation in your legs.

8. Mood Swings and Emotional Changes

Hormonal changes, fatigue, and the physical demands of pregnancy can lead to emotional ups and downs.

- **Mindfulness and Meditation**: Practicing mindfulness or meditation can help manage stress and improve emotional well-being.

- **Prenatal Yoga**: Yoga not only helps with physical discomfort but can also improve mental clarity and reduce anxiety.

- **Talk About Your Feelings**: Share your thoughts and emotions with friends, family, or a healthcare provider. Joining a support group for pregnant women can also help you connect with others experiencing similar feelings.

9. Skin Changes (Itching, Stretch Marks)

Many women experience skin changes during pregnancy, such as itching, stretch marks, or increased sensitivity.

- **Moisturise**: Use natural oils or creams with ingredients like cocoa butter, shea butter, or vitamin E to keep the skin hydrated and reduce the risk of stretch marks.

- **Oatmeal Baths**: For itching, taking an oatmeal bath can soothe the skin.

- **Stay Hydrated**: Drink plenty of water to keep your skin hydrated from within.

- **Wear Sunscreen**: Pregnancy can increase skin sensitivity, so always use a safe, natural sunscreen to prevent dark spots and protect your skin.

- **Ensure adequate Omega 3 and Zinc**: Both of these can help keep your skin healthy and prevent stretch marks. Your pre-natal may have enough zinc but do check and discuss this with your healthcare provider.

10. Insomnia

Many pregnant women have trouble sleeping due to physical discomfort or anxiety.

- **Establish a Relaxing Bedtime Routine**: A warm bath, reading, or meditation before bed can help you relax and improve sleep quality.

- **Sleep on Your Left Side**: Sleeping on your left side can improve circulation and reduce pressure on your back and major blood vessels.

- **Use Pillows for Support**: Use a pregnancy pillow or extra pillows to support your belly, back, and knees.

- **Limit Caffeine**: Avoid caffeine later in the day to improve sleep quality.

General Tips for a Healthy Pregnancy

- **Stay Active**: Regular exercise (with your doctor's approval) can help reduce pregnancy discomforts, improve mood, and support overall health.

- **Stay Hydrated**: Proper hydration is essential for healthy blood flow, digestion, and managing pregnancy symptoms.

- **Balanced Diet**: Eat a diet rich in whole foods like fruits, vegetables, lean proteins, whole grains, and healthy fats to support your body and your growing baby.

- **Take Prenatal Vitamins**: Ensure you're getting the necessary vitamins and minerals, particularly folic acid, iron, calcium, and DHA, which are important for both maternal and foetal health.

By incorporating these natural remedies and lifestyle changes, many women can experience relief from common pregnancy symptoms and enjoy a healthier, more comfortable pregnancy. However, it's always important to consult with a healthcare provider before trying any new remedies or supplements.

Conclusion:

Preparing for pregnancy is about more than just conception; it's about creating the healthiest possible environment for both you and your future baby. By understanding the process of folliculogenesis and creating a healthy egg, taking steps to detoxify your body and ensuring the best environment for your growing baby, will ensure a happy and healthy child is born.

Chapter 15

Preparing for Childbirth: What to Expect and How to Get Ready

Introduction: The Journey to Childbirth

Childbirth is one of the most profound and transformative experiences in life. Whether you're preparing for your first child or adding another member to your family, the anticipation and uncertainty of labour and delivery can be both exciting and overwhelming. Understanding what to expect, how to prepare, and what both the ideal and less-than-ideal scenarios might look like can help ease anxieties and ensure that you and your partner are as ready as possible for the arrival of your baby.

This chapter will guide you through the key aspects of preparing for childbirth, from practical preparations and birthing plans to mental and emotional readiness. We'll explore both the best-case and worst-case scenarios, offering strategies to prepare for each. Additionally, we'll discuss how both mom and dad can actively participate in the process, ensuring a supportive and collaborative experience.

Understanding Childbirth: The Basics

Braxton Hicks: I'm sure you've seen these on TV or in movies! Braxton Hicks contractions, also known as practice contractions or false labour, are sporadic uterine contractions that may start around six weeks into a pregnancy. However, they are usually felt in the second or third trimester of pregnancy. They are perfectly normal, but future parents will often find themselves at the hospital when they are first experienced. Don't panic, you won't be the first person who does this, and the hospital staff will be sympathetic.

Once true labour starts, Childbirth typically occurs in three stages:

1. **Stage 1: Labour**

     o   **Early Labour:** The cervix begins to dilate and efface (thin out). Contractions start but are usually mild and irregular.

     o   **Active Labour:** The cervix dilates more rapidly, contractions become stronger, more regular, and closer together. This phase can last several hours and is different for each woman and each pregnancy. Stress is not a good things at this point because adrenaline antagonises (stops it from working) Oxytocin, which is the labour hormone. If you are stressed, focus on breathing if you can.

- o **Transition:** The final part of active labour, where the cervix completes dilation to 10 centimetres. This is often the most intense part of labour.

2. **Stage 2: Delivery of the Baby**

   - o Pushing begins once the cervix is fully dilated, and the baby is delivered through the birth canal.

3. **Stage 3: Delivery of the Placenta**

   - o After the baby is born, contractions will continue to help deliver the placenta, usually within 5 to 30 minutes after the birth. This step is never shown in movies and can take unprepared new mothers by surprise!

Preparing for Childbirth: Practical Steps

1. Choosing Your Birth Setting and Team

- **Hospital Birth:** Most women choose to give birth in a hospital where there is access to medical interventions if needed. Discuss with your healthcare provider the hospital's policies and what options (such as epidurals or birth pools) are available.

- **Birth Centre:** A middle ground between home and hospital, birth centres often provide a more homelike environment with a focus on natural birth, while still having medical staff available.

- **Home Birth:** For those seeking a natural, familiar setting, home birth may be an option, usually attended by a midwife. It's important to have a backup plan in case a transfer to a hospital becomes necessary.

2. Creating a Birth Plan

- A birth plan is a document that outlines your preferences for labour, delivery, and postpartum care. It might include your wishes regarding pain management, who you want present during birth, whether you plan to breastfeed immediately after delivery, and any specific requests you have about the birth environment.

- Keep in mind that while it's good to have a plan, flexibility is essential. Childbirth can be unpredictable, and being open to adjustments can help you stay calm and focused.

3. Packing Your Hospital Bag

- **For Mom:**
  - Comfortable clothing (such as a robe and loose-fitting pants)
  - Slippers and socks
  - Toiletries (toothbrush, hairbrush, lip balm, etc.)
  - Maternity pads and nursing bras

- o   Snacks and drinks for energy
- o   Important documents (ID, insurance information, birth plan)

- **For Baby:**
  - o   Newborn clothing (onesies, socks, hat)
  - o   Swaddle blanket
  - o   Diapers/nappies and wipes
  - o   Car seat for the ride home

- **For Dad/Partner:**
  - o   Comfortable clothes
  - o   Snacks and drinks
  - o   Camera or phone for pictures
  - o   Toiletries and any medications

4. Prenatal Classes and Education

- Attending childbirth classes can help demystify the process and build confidence. These classes often cover topics such as breathing techniques, stages of labour, pain management options, and postpartum care.

- Consider also taking classes on newborn care, breastfeeding, and infant CPR to feel more prepared once the baby arrives.

5. Mental and Emotional Preparation

- **Visualisation and Positive Affirmations:** Practice visualising a smooth labour and delivery. Positive affirmations can help build a mindset of strength and calmness.

- **Communication with Your Partner:** Ensure that you and your partner discuss expectations, fears, and roles during labour. This can prevent misunderstandings and foster a stronger bond during the experience.

- **Mindfulness and Relaxation Techniques:** Techniques such as deep breathing, meditation, and progressive muscle relaxation can help manage pain and reduce anxiety during labour.

What to Expect: The Ideal Scenario

In an ideal scenario, labour progresses smoothly, the baby is born without complications, and both mother and baby are healthy. Here's what you might expect in this best-case scenario:

1. **Labour Starts Naturally:** Contractions begin gradually and increase in intensity. The baby is in a favourable position, and the cervix dilates at a steady pace.

2. **Effective Pain Management:** Whether you choose natural pain relief methods (like breathing exercises,

water immersion, heat packs or massage) or medical options (such as an epidural), your pain is manageable and allows you to focus on the birth.

3. **Supportive Birth Team:** Your partner, healthcare providers, and any other support persons are present, attentive, and respectful of your birth plan.

4. **Healthy Delivery:** The baby is born vaginally without complications. Skin-to-skin contact is initiated immediately, and the baby starts breastfeeding within the first hour.

5. **Smooth Postpartum Recovery:** The placenta is delivered without issue, and bleeding is within normal limits. Both mother and baby receive necessary postpartum care, and you feel supported as you begin recovery.

Preparing for Less-Than-Ideal Scenarios

While it's natural to hope for the best, it's important to prepare for potential challenges. These might include:

1. Labour Complications

- **Prolonged Labour:** Sometimes, labour stalls or progresses very slowly, which can be exhausting and frustrating. If this happens, your healthcare provider may suggest interventions such as breaking your water, administering Pitocin (a drug to stimulate contractions), or considering a C-section.

- **Foetal Distress:** If the baby shows signs of distress (such as abnormal heart rates), your medical team may recommend interventions like oxygen for the mother, changing your position, or in some cases, an emergency C-section.

2. Unexpected Delivery Complications

- **Emergency C-Section:** If a vaginal delivery is not possible or safe, a C-section may be performed. While this can be a surprising turn of events, knowing that this is a possibility can help you mentally prepare. If you do have a C-section, consider vaginal seeding. Vaginal seeding is the practice of wiping a baby's mouth, face and skin with its mother's vaginal fluids after C-section. This process transfers vaginal microbes to the baby to help establish the baby's own microbiome to promote good health and fight disease.

- **Assisted Delivery:** Tools such as forceps or a vacuum may be used if the baby needs help passing through the birth canal. These interventions can be necessary for the safety of both mother and baby.

3. Postpartum Challenges

- **Heavy Bleeding:** Postpartum haemorrhage is a rare but serious condition. Your healthcare team will monitor you closely after birth, but being aware of the symptoms can help you act quickly if needed.

- **Breastfeeding Difficulties:** Some new mothers struggle with breastfeeding due to latch issues, low milk supply, or pain. Lactation consultants can provide valuable support in these situations.

How Both Parents Can Prepare

1. For Mom:

- **Physical Preparation:** Regular prenatal exercise (with your doctor's approval) can help build stamina for labour. Activities like walking, swimming, or prenatal yoga can strengthen muscles and improve flexibility.

- **Nutritional Support:** A balanced diet rich in nutrients supports both your health and your baby's development. Focus on protein, healthy fats, complex carbohydrates, and plenty of fruits and vegetables. Stay hydrated and consider prenatal vitamins as recommended by your healthcare provider.

- **Emotional Preparation:** Address any fears or anxieties you may have. Talking with other moms, joining support groups, or speaking with a counsellor can provide reassurance and reduce stress.

2. For Dad/Partner:

- **Education:** Attend prenatal classes with your partner to understand what to expect during labour and delivery. Knowledge of the stages of labour, pain management options, and ways to support your partner can make you an invaluable part of the birth team.

- **Practical Support:** Be prepared to assist with tasks like timing contractions, helping with relaxation techniques, and advocating for your partner's preferences during labour.

- **Emotional Support:** Your calm, reassuring presence can make a big difference. Be ready to offer encouragement, physical comfort (like holding hands or providing a massage), and emotional support throughout the process.

Conclusion:

Childbirth is a powerful experience that marks the beginning of a new chapter in your life. While it's impossible to predict exactly how your labour and delivery will unfold, being well-prepared can help you face the journey with confidence and resilience.

Remember that every birth is unique. Whether everything goes according to plan, or you face unexpected challenges, the most important outcome is the health and well-being of both mother and baby. By taking the time to educate yourselves, create a supportive environment, and prepare both mentally and physically, you and your partner will be ready to welcome your baby into the world with open arms.

Chapter 16

The Postpartum Period: Recovery, Bonding, and Navigating Early Parenthood

Introduction: Entering the Postpartum Period

The postpartum period, often referred to as the "fourth trimester," is a time of significant physical, emotional, and psychological change. After the intense experience of childbirth, new parents embark on the journey of early parenthood, which is filled with both challenges and joys. This chapter will guide you through the postpartum recovery process, the importance of bonding with your baby, and practical strategies to navigate the early days of parenthood.

We'll explore how to care for your body as it heals, the emotional shifts that may occur, and how to establish a strong bond with your newborn. Additionally, we'll discuss the importance of self-care, support systems, and realistic expectations as you adjust to life with your new baby.

Postpartum Recovery: Healing Your Body

1. Physical Recovery After Vaginal Birth

- **Vaginal Soreness:** It's common to experience soreness or discomfort around the perineum, especially if you had a tear or episiotomy. Using cold packs, sitting on a cushion, and keeping the area clean can help with healing.

- **Lochia:** After childbirth, your body will shed the lining of the uterus, which appears as vaginal discharge known as lochia. This bleeding can last for several weeks and gradually lightens from bright red to pink, then white or yellow.

- **Breast Engorgement:** As your milk comes in, your breasts may become swollen and tender. Frequent breastfeeding or pumping, wearing a supportive bra, and applying warm compresses can help relieve discomfort.

- **Postpartum Cramps:** Also known as afterpains, these cramps occur as your uterus contracts back to its pre-pregnancy size. They are often more noticeable during breastfeeding due to the release of oxytocin.

- **Day 3 Rage:** It's normal, your hormones are fluctuating wildly, and many women experience anger/rage around this day. It is important for both parents to be mentally prepared for this to happen and manage it for what it is, the rapid change in hormones after birth, NOT the husbands loud chewing (unless it is, then chew quieter!).

2. Physical Recovery After Caesarean Section

- **Incision Care:** Keep the incision site clean and dry, and watch for signs of infection such as redness, swelling, or discharge. Follow your doctor's instructions on caring for the wound.

- **Movement and Rest:** Gentle movement, like short walks, can aid in recovery and prevent complications like blood clots. However, avoid strenuous activity and lifting heavy objects until your doctor gives the green light.

- **Managing Pain:** Pain management is crucial in the days following a C-section. Follow your doctor's recommendations for pain relief, which may include prescribed medications or over-the-counter options.

3. Pelvic Floor Recovery

- **Kegel Exercises:** Strengthening the pelvic floor muscles through Kegel exercises can help improve bladder control and support the healing process. Start gently and gradually increase the intensity as your body heals.

- **Pelvic Physical Therapy:** If you experience ongoing issues like incontinence, pain during intercourse, or pelvic organ prolapse, consider consulting a pelvic floor physical therapist for targeted exercises and treatment.

4. Postpartum Nutrition and Hydration

- **Nutrient-Dense Diet:** Your body needs adequate nutrition to heal and support breastfeeding. Focus on a diet rich in lean proteins, whole grains, fruits, vegetables, and healthy fats. Consider foods high in zinc, iron, calcium, and fibre to support recovery and energy levels. Continue taking your prenatal nutrients until you stop breastfeeding.

- **Hydration:** Staying hydrated is crucial, especially if you're breastfeeding. Drink plenty of water throughout the day and consider herbal teas or broths to increase fluid intake.

- **Supplements:** Continue taking prenatal vitamins during the postpartum period to ensure you're getting essential nutrients like zinc, iron, vitamin D, and folic acid (folate).

Bonding with Your Baby: Building a Strong Connection

1. Skin-to-Skin Contact

- **The Importance of Skin-to-Skin with both parents:** It is important for BOTH parents to do this. Holding your baby close, skin-to-skin, immediately after birth and in the days following can regulate their heart rate, temperature, and breathing. It also promotes bonding and helps with breastfeeding initiation.

- **How to Practice:** Lay your baby on your chest with their bare skin against yours. This can be done during feeding, while they are awake, or even when they're sleeping.

2. Breastfeeding and Bonding

- **Breastfeeding Benefits:** Breastfeeding is not only about nutrition; it's a key bonding activity. The release of oxytocin during breastfeeding helps strengthen the emotional connection between mother and baby.

- **Challenges and Support:** Breastfeeding doesn't always come naturally. If you face challenges, seek support from a lactation consultant, your healthcare provider, or breastfeeding support groups.

3. Responding to Cues

- **Understanding Baby's Signals:** Newborns communicate through cries, facial expressions, and body language. Learning to recognise and respond to these cues builds trust and security, fostering a strong bond.

- **Comforting Your Baby:** Holding, rocking, singing, and speaking softly to your baby can soothe them when they're distressed and strengthen your bond.

4. Involving Dad/Partner in Bonding

- **Shared Activities:** Encourage your partner to participate in skin-to-skin contact, diaper changes, bath time, and soothing activities. These moments create a bond between the baby and the non-birthing parent.

- **Supporting Breastfeeding:** Partners can support breastfeeding by bringing the baby to the mother, helping with positioning, or simply offering encouragement and support.

Navigating Early Parenthood: Challenges and Joys

1. Emotional Changes and Mental Health

- **Baby Blues:** It's common for new mothers to experience mood swings, irritability, and sadness in the first couple of weeks after birth, known as the "baby blues." This is due to hormonal changes, exhaustion, and the overwhelming nature of new parenthood.

- **Postpartum Depression:** If feelings of sadness, anxiety, or hopelessness persist or worsen, it may be postpartum depression. This condition is serious but treatable with professional help. Don't hesitate to reach out to a healthcare provider if you're struggling. Adequate zinc during your pregnancy has been shown to reduce stretch marks as well as reduce the risk of postnatal depression.

- **Supporting Your Partner:** Both parents can experience emotional shifts. Open communication and mutual support are vital during this time. If one partner is struggling, seeking help together can be beneficial.

2. Establishing Routines

- **Feeding Schedule:** Newborns often feed every 2-3 hours, whether breastfed or formula-fed. Establishing a feeding routine can help regulate your baby's hunger cues and ensure they're getting enough nourishment.

- **Sleep Patterns:** Newborns sleep a lot but in short intervals. Understanding your baby's sleep patterns and creating a calm sleep environment can help everyone get the rest they need.

- **Self-Care for Parents:** While routines focus on the baby, self-care for parents is equally important. Try to prioritize your own sleep, nutrition, and mental health. Accept help from family and friends, and don't hesitate to ask for assistance.

3. Handling Common Newborn Challenges

- **Crying:** It's normal for babies to cry, and sometimes the cause isn't immediately clear. Checking for basic needs (hunger, diaper change, comfort) and offering soothing techniques can help calm your baby.

- **Colic:** If your baby cries excessively and seems inconsolable, they may have colic. While this phase is challenging, it usually resolves by 3-4 months. Holding your baby upright, swaddling, and using white noise may help.

- **Diapering and Bathing:** These basic care tasks can take time to master. Practice patience and gentleness, and soon these routines will become second nature.

4. Adjusting to New Family Dynamics

- **Communicating with Your Partner:** The arrival of a baby can strain even the strongest relationships. Maintain open lines of communication, share parenting responsibilities, and check in with each other regularly.

- **Managing Visitors and Support:** While it's wonderful to have support from family and friends, it's okay to set boundaries to protect your time and space. Prioritize what's best for your recovery and your new family.

- **Sibling Adjustment:** If you have other children, involve them in caring for the new baby. Acknowledge their feelings and spend quality time with them to ease the transition.

5. Celebrating the Joys

- **Firsts:** Cherish the small milestones, your baby's first smile, the first time they grasp your finger, the first time they sleep through the night. These moments are fleeting and precious.

- **Parenting Achievements:** Recognise and celebrate your successes as parents. Whether it's mastering a new skill or surviving a tough day, each accomplishment is a step forward in your parenting journey.

- **Building Memories:** Take time to enjoy these early days. Capture moments with photos, keep a journal, or simply Savor the quiet times when you can hold your baby close.

Conclusion:

The postpartum period is a time of immense change and growth. While it comes with its share of challenges, it's also a time of deep bonding, personal transformation, and the beginning of your journey as a parent. By focusing on recovery, building a strong connection with your baby, and navigating the ups and downs of early parenthood with patience and resilience, you can create a positive and fulfilling experience for both you and your new family.

Chapter 17

Understanding Perimenopause: Navigating Puberty in Reverse

Perimenopause, is like reverse puberty and is often referred to as the transition phase leading up to menopause and is a significant period in a woman's life marked by fluctuating hormone levels. This phase can begin in the early 40s or even late 30s and typically lasts for several years until menopause, which is defined as 12 consecutive months without a menstrual period. Understanding perimenopause is crucial for managing its symptoms and maintaining quality of life during this transition.

In this chapter, we will explore the hormonal changes that occur during perimenopause, the common symptoms women experience, and the various approaches to managing these symptoms. We'll discuss conventional treatments like Hormone Replacement Therapy (HRT), including bioidentical and body-identical hormones, as well as naturopathic strategies that can support this transition. Remember that the basics, such as good gut health, stress management, sleep and exercise should always be covered to ensure a healthy transition.

The Hormonal Changes During Perimenopause

Perimenopause is characterised by a gradual decline in ovarian function, which leads to fluctuations in the levels of key hormones such as oestrogen, progesterone, and testosterone. Understanding these changes is essential for grasping the symptoms and treatment options available.

1. Oestrogen

- **Fluctuating Levels:** During perimenopause, oestrogen levels can be unpredictable, sometimes soaring and other times plummeting. This fluctuation can cause irregular periods, hot flashes, and mood swings. This is caused by the ovaries slowing down their overall production of the hormones.

- **Dominance AND Deficiency:** This is where things get confusing, because, in the early stages of perimenopause, women might experience periods of oestrogen dominance (where oestrogen is high relative to progesterone if they don't ovulate) which can lead to symptoms like moodiness, heavy periods and breast tenderness, as well as the symptoms of deficiency as the overall levels decline, contributing to additional symptoms like vaginal dryness and night sweats.

2. Progesterone

- **Decline in Production:** Progesterone levels begin to decline earlier than oestrogen during perimenopause, often leading to an imbalance between the two hormones called oestrogen dominance. This can result in symptoms like anxiety, insomnia, and irregular menstrual cycles.

- **Impact on Sleep and Mood:** Progesterone has a calming effect on the brain and promotes sleep. As levels drop, many women experience increased anxiety, anger and sleep disturbances. These symptoms can be scary when they come first arrive, especially if the women wasn't prepared for them!

3. Testosterone

- **Gradual Decline:** Although testosterone is often associated with men, it plays a vital role in women's health as well. During perimenopause, testosterone levels decline, which can lead to decreased libido, fatigue, and reduced muscle mass.

- **Influence on Energy and Libido:** Testosterone contributes to overall energy levels, motivation, and sexual desire. As levels decrease, women may notice a reduction in these areas.

Common Symptoms of Perimenopause

The hormonal fluctuations during perimenopause can lead to a wide range of symptoms, which vary in severity from woman to woman. Recognising these symptoms is the first step toward effective management.

1. Irregular Periods

- **Changes in Cycle Length:** Women may notice their menstrual cycles becoming shorter or longer. Some may experience missed periods, while others have heavier or lighter bleeding.

- **Spotting and Clotting:** Spotting between periods or clotting during menstruation can also occur due to hormonal imbalances.

2. Hot Flashes and Night Sweats

- **Sudden Warmth:** Hot flashes, a hallmark of perimenopause, involve sudden feelings of warmth, often followed by sweating and chills. They can occur during the day or night, leading to night sweats that disrupt sleep.

- **Triggers and Management:** Stress, caffeine, alcohol, and spicy foods can trigger hot flashes. Managing these triggers, dressing in layers, and using cooling strategies can help alleviate symptoms.

3. Sleep Disturbances

- **Difficulty Falling Asleep:** Many women find it harder to fall asleep or stay asleep during perimenopause due to hormonal changes, particularly the decline in progesterone.

- **Night Sweats and Insomnia:** Night sweats can wake women from sleep, contributing to insomnia and daytime fatigue.

4. Mood Swings and Anxiety

- **Emotional Rollercoaster:** The hormonal fluctuations of perimenopause can lead to mood swings, irritability, and anxiety. Some women may also experience symptoms of depression. These symptoms are much worse if a woman hasn't addressed her adrenal health leading up to the changes.

- **Brain Fog:** Difficulty concentrating and forgetfulness, often referred to as "brain fog," are also common during perimenopause.

5. Vaginal Dryness and Changes in Libido

- **Decreased Oestrogen:** As oestrogen levels decline, vaginal tissues can become thinner, drier, and less elastic, leading to discomfort during intercourse.

- **Impact on Sexual Health:** Many women report a decrease in libido during perimenopause, influenced by hormonal changes, stress, and other symptoms like fatigue.

- **Changes in the vaginal microbiome:** The changes in oestrogen levels can impact the vaginal microbiome, leading to pain, itchiness and an increase in the frequency of urinary tract infections. You can test this microbiome and use probiotics to rebalance it if needed.

6. Weight Gain and Metabolic Changes

- **Slower Metabolism:** Hormonal changes can slow metabolism, leading to weight gain, especially around the abdomen. This is annoying, but, when your ovaries can no longer make oestrogen, what happens is that testosterone in your fatty tissue is aromatised into oestrogen. So having a little bit of extra weight in perimenopause is not the end of the world and it generally leaves once fully in menopause if you eat right, sleep well, exercise and don't stress too much. Hashimoto's can also be triggered by the stages of oestrogen dominance, so keep an eye on your adrenals and thyroid markers.

- **Insulin Resistance:** Some women may develop insulin resistance during perimenopause, making it more challenging to maintain a healthy weight. This is more of an issue and needs to be addressed through a change of diet, exercise and possibly supplementing something like Berberine to manage your sugar and insulin levels. Many women benefit from wearing a continuous glucose monitor during this stage to see how their body is responding to food and adjusting to their own unique metabolic needs. Chat with your healthcare provider if you feel like this may help.

Allergies and Perimenopause:

During perimenopause and with the use of hormone replacement therapy (HRT), allergies and histamine responses may worsen due to changes in hormone levels, particularly oestrogen. Here's how it works:

1. Oestrogen Increases Histamine Release

Oestrogen plays a significant role in the immune system and influences the release of histamine, a chemical that causes allergy symptoms like itching, swelling, and inflammation.

Histamine Release: Oestrogen can stimulate mast cells, which are immune cells responsible for releasing histamine.

Higher oestrogen levels cause these cells to release more histamine, leading to worsened allergy symptoms.

Histamine Degradation: Oestrogen also reduces the activity of an enzyme called **diamine oxidase (DAO)**, which is responsible for breaking down histamine. As a result, histamine lingers in the body longer, worsening allergy symptoms.

2. Fluctuating Oestrogen Levels During Perimenopause

Perimenopause is marked by irregular and fluctuating levels of oestrogen. This inconsistency can make histamine release unpredictable, triggering or worsening allergic reactions.

Higher Oestrogen Phases: When oestrogen spikes during this period, it can lead to an increase in histamine production, causing more severe allergy symptoms, including hay fever, asthma, and even skin reactions like hives.

3. Impact of Hormone Replacement Therapy (HRT)

HRT often involves oestrogen or a combination of oestrogen and progesterone to relieve menopausal symptoms.

Oestrogen HRT: If a woman starts taking oestrogen as part of HRT, this can elevate histamine levels, exacerbating allergies or making women more sensitive to allergens.

Progesterone's Role: Progesterone can have a stabilising effect on mast cells, helping to counteract the histamine-releasing effect of oestrogen. However, in some cases, imbalances in HRT (such as not enough progesterone) can still worsen allergies.

4. Lower Progesterone Levels During Perimenopause

In perimenopause, progesterone levels generally decline before oestrogen levels do. Progesterone helps stabilise mast cells, so when its levels drop, there may be less control over histamine release, leading to an increase in allergic reactions.

5. Cross-Reactivity with Histamine Intolerance

Some women may also experience **histamine intolerance** during perimenopause or with HRT. This is a condition where the body accumulates excess histamine and cannot break it down efficiently, which can cause symptoms like headaches, flushing, and worsened allergies. The combination of fluctuating oestrogen levels and histamine intolerance can make these symptoms more pronounced.

If you are experiencing histamine issues, binders (like clay and charcoal) have been shown to bind to excess histamine in the gut and can help reduce the overall load.

Managing Perimenopause Symptoms

Effective management of perimenopause symptoms often requires a combination of approaches, tailored to the individual. A holistic approach, integrating conventional treatments like HRT with lifestyle modifications and naturopathic strategies works wonders.

1. Hormone Replacement Therapy (HRT)

- **Traditional HRT:** This involves using synthetic hormones to replace the oestrogen, progesterone and testosterone that the body no longer produces in adequate amounts. It can be highly effective in relieving symptoms like hot flashes, night sweats, and vaginal dryness.

- **Bioidentical Hormone Replacement Therapy (BHRT):** BHRT uses hormones that are chemically identical to those produced by the human body. These are often derived from plant sources and are customized based on an individual's hormonal needs, usually determined through blood or saliva testing.

- **Body-Identical HRT:** This refers to hormones that are identical in structure to endogenous hormones and are often prescribed in standard doses available on the market. They are similar to bioidentical hormones but are not custom-compounded.

- **Benefits and Risks:** HRT can significantly improve quality of life for women experiencing severe perimenopause symptoms. However, it's important to discuss the risks and benefits with a healthcare provider, as HRT is not suitable for everyone, particularly those with a history of certain cancers or blood clots.

2. Naturopathic Approaches

- **Diet and Nutrition:**
  - **Phytoestrogens:** Incorporating foods rich in phytoestrogens, such as flaxseeds, soy, and legumes, can help balance oestrogen levels naturally. They won't increase the oestrogen but bind to the receptor sites and can help with symptoms. If you are no longer making oestrogen, then it will need to be replaced and you will need to talk to a prescriber who can help you.

  - **Anti-Inflammatory Diet:** An anti-inflammatory diet rich in fruits, vegetables, whole grains, and omega-3 fatty acids can help manage symptoms like joint pain, weight gain, and mood swings.

  - **Supplementation:** Certain supplements, such as magnesium for sleep and anxiety, B vitamins for energy and mood, and omega-3s for brain health, can support women during perimenopause. Electrolytes are often overlooked and depleted in this life stage thanks to the stress leading up to it and that it causes, so please also consider replacing your electrolytes.

- **Herbal Remedies:**
  - **Black Cohosh:** Known for its potential to reduce hot flashes and night sweats.
  - **Vitex (Chaste Tree Berry):** Supports progesterone production and may help with menstrual irregularities and mood swings.
  - **Ashwagandha:** An adaptogen that helps the body manage stress and balance hormones.
  - **Quercetin:** This flavanol, along with Vitamin C, can help with the histamine issues.
  - **Korean herbs:** Cynanchum wilfordii, Angelica Gigas, Phlomis umbrosa, have been shown to have a synergistic effect when combined and can reduce most of the main symptoms associated with menopause.
  - **ERr 731°:** A plant-based and hormone-free ingredient clinically proven to relieve 12 of the most common symptoms of menopause by up to 83%. Its proprietary non oestrogen formula works with a woman's body to bring you back into balance naturally.

- **Lifestyle Modifications:**

    - **Exercise:** Regular physical activity, particularly strength training and aerobic exercise, can improve mood, support weight management, and enhance overall well-being.

    - **Stress Management:** Practices like yoga, meditation, and deep breathing exercises can reduce stress and help manage perimenopausal symptoms.

    - **Sleep Hygiene:** Creating a sleep-friendly environment, maintaining a regular sleep schedule, and limiting caffeine and screen time before bed can improve sleep quality.

3. Integrative Approaches

- **Acupuncture:** Some women find relief from perimenopausal symptoms through acupuncture, which can help balance hormones and reduce stress.

- **Functional Medicine:** This approach involves a comprehensive evaluation of hormonal health, lifestyle, and nutrition, followed by personalised treatment plans that may include dietary changes, supplements, and bioidentical hormones.

4. I3C vs DIM 3 in managing Oestrogen Dominance in perimenopause.

Indole-3-Carbinol (I3C) and Diindolylmethane (DIM) both play a role in balancing oestrogen in perimenopause. They work specifically is reducing oestrogen, so it is important in this stage of your hormone balancing, to understand when it is relevant to take them or not. As they both reduce oestrogen from circulation, only use them if you are definitely oestrogen dominant and have the relevant symptoms. Do not take them if you are oestrogen deficient. Use sulforaphane instead, this will help detoxification without reducing your circulating oestrogen.

Both **Indole-3-carbinol (I3C)** and **Diindolylmethane (DIM)** are compounds found in cruciferous vegetables like broccoli, Brussels sprouts, cabbage, and kale, and both are known for their roles in oestrogen metabolism. However, they differ in their structure, how they are processed in the body, and their specific effects on oestrogen detoxification. Here's a breakdown of the key differences and their roles in oestrogen metabolism:

1. Chemical Structure and Source

- **Indole-3-Carbinol (I3C):** I3C is a precursor compound found in raw cruciferous vegetables. It is not stable in the acidic environment of the stomach, where it undergoes rapid conversion into various compounds, including DIM.

- **Diindolylmethane (DIM):** DIM is the main bioactive compound derived from I3C. When I3C is ingested, it forms DIM as one of its primary metabolites in the digestive process.

2. Formation

- **I3C:** When you consume cruciferous vegetables, I3C is released and then converted into DIM and other metabolites during digestion. It needs good stomach acid to convert to DIM and many people don't have the best acid and may need to add HCL when taking the I3C. I3C itself is rarely active in its original form due to its instability.

- **DIM:** This compound is already in its bioactive form, and once I3C is metabolized into DIM, it becomes more stable and exerts its effects on oestrogen metabolism.

3. Role in Oestrogen Detoxification/Metabolism

Both I3C and DIM play crucial roles in oestrogen detoxification and metabolism, particularly by influencing the balance of oestrogen metabolites. Oestrogen is metabolised through different pathways, producing various metabolites that can have either protective or harmful effects in the body.

I3C:

- **Influences Phase I Detoxification (CYP Enzymes):** I3C promotes the activity of cytochrome P450 (CYP) enzymes, especially CYP1A1 and CYP1B1, which are involved in oestrogen metabolism. It helps shift oestrogen metabolism towards the formation of **2-hydroxyestrone (2-OHE1)**, a "good" oestrogen metabolite with weaker estrogenic activity, and away from **16-alpha-hydroxyestrone (16α-OHE1)**, which has stronger, potentially harmful effects, including promoting cell proliferation and increasing cancer risk.

- **Protects against Oestrogen Dominance:** By influencing these pathways, I3C helps reduce the risk of oestrogen dominance, which is linked to conditions like breast cancer and endometriosis.

DIM:

- **Supports Phase II Detoxification:** DIM enhances oestrogen metabolism by promoting the breakdown of oestrogen into beneficial metabolites, specifically the 2-hydroxyestrone (2-OHE1) pathway. This pathway results in the production of metabolites that have anti-estrogenic and anti-carcinogenic properties.

- **Oestrogen Receptor Modulation:** DIM acts as a selective oestrogen receptor modulator (SERM), meaning it can exert both estrogenic and anti-estrogenic effects depending on the tissue. This helps balance oestrogen levels and reduce the risk of oestrogen-related cancers.

- **Anti-inflammatory and Anti-carcinogenic Effects:** Besides oestrogen metabolism, DIM has been found to reduce inflammation and has anti-tumour properties, especially in hormone-sensitive tissues like the breast, uterus, and prostate.

4. Health Benefits and Uses

Both I3C and DIM are used for their potential health benefits, especially in women's health and hormone balance. However, they have different applications:

- **I3C:** It is used primarily for its broader impact on detoxification and oestrogen metabolism. It has been researched for its potential role in cancer prevention, particularly breast and cervical cancers. However, I3C is less commonly taken as a supplement due to its conversion into multiple metabolites (including DIM), making its effects less predictable.

- **DIM:** DIM is more commonly used in supplement form for hormone balance, particularly for managing oestrogen dominance, premenstrual syndrome (PMS), polycystic ovary syndrome (PCOS), and menopausal symptoms. Its effects on promoting favourable oestrogen metabolism make it a popular choice for women's hormone health. However, it may not be suitable in the later stages of peri menopause when oestrogen levels are dropping, so please consult with a healthcare provider if you are considering this at this stage of life.

Summary of Differences

Aspect	Indole-3-Carbinol (I3C)	Diindolylmethane (DIM)
Source	Found in cruciferous vegetables	Metabolite of I3C
Stability	Unstable, converts to DIM and other compounds	More stable and bioactive
Main Role	Influences Phase I detox, promotes 2-OHE1 production	Supports Phase II detox, promotes 2-OHE1 production
Mechanism	Induces CYP enzymes for oestrogen metabolism	Modulates oestrogen receptors, promotes "good" oestrogens
Supplement Form	Less commonly used as a standalone supplement	More commonly used for oestrogen balance
Health Focus	Broader detoxification, cancer prevention potential	Hormone balance, oestrogen dominance management

Conclusion:

Perimenopause is a natural phase of life, but it can be challenging due to the wide range of symptoms and hormonal changes. By understanding what's happening in your body and exploring the various treatment options, you can navigate this transition with greater ease and confidence.

A personalised approach, combining conventional and naturopathic strategies to manage symptoms and maintain quality of life. Whether you choose HRT, bioidentical hormones, or natural remedies, the key is to find what works best for you and to seek support from healthcare providers who understand the complexities of perimenopause.

As you move through perimenopause, remember that this is a time of transformation. With the right tools and knowledge, you can embrace this phase of life with resilience, grace, and a renewed focus on your health and well-being.

Chapter 18

Embracing Menopause:

Caring for Your Brain, Bones, and Heart

Introduction: A New Chapter in Life

Menopause is a significant milestone in a woman's life, marking the end of menstrual cycles and the transition into a new phase of maturity. While this natural process is often accompanied by a mix of emotions—relief for some, anxiety for others—it's important to understand that menopause is not just about the end of fertility. It also brings profound changes to your body, particularly affecting the brain, bones, and cardiovascular system.

This chapter is designed to provide you with a caring, supportive perspective on menopause, focusing on how these changes occur and what you can do to protect your health. We'll explore how menopause impacts your brain, bones, and heart, and offer practical strategies to help you mitigate these effects and maintain your well-being.

Understanding Menopause: What's Happening in Your Body?

Menopause is defined as the time when a woman has gone 12 consecutive months without a menstrual period, typically occurring between the ages of 45 and 55, although many women go through premature ovarian failure as young as in their twenties and others can continue menstruating into their 60's. Surgical menopause occurs when the uterus and ovaries are surgically removed.

The years leading up to menopause, known as perimenopause, involve significant hormonal fluctuations, particularly in oestrogen and progesterone levels. As these hormones decline, they trigger a cascade of changes in various systems of the body.

The Brain: Cognitive and Emotional Changes

Oestrogen plays a crucial role in brain function, influencing mood, memory, and cognitive abilities. As oestrogen levels decline during menopause, many women experience changes in their mental and emotional well-being.

- **Memory and Cognitive Function:** Some women notice increased forgetfulness, difficulty concentrating, and a phenomenon commonly referred to as "brain fog." While these cognitive changes can be frustrating, they are typically mild and often improve over time. Adrenal health and chronic low grade inflammation can make this worse and these root causes should be addressed to improve the health of the brain.

- **Mood and Mental Health:** The decline in oestrogen can also impact neurotransmitters like serotonin, which regulates mood. As a result, some women experience mood swings, anxiety, or even depression during menopause. These emotional changes can be compounded by life stressors, making it essential to address them with care and compassion.

- **Sleep Disturbances:** Hot flashes and night sweats, common symptoms of menopause, can disrupt sleep, further affecting cognitive function and mood. Poor sleep quality can exacerbate feelings of fatigue and irritability.

The Bones: Protecting Your Skeletal Health

Oestrogen and testosterone are both vital for maintaining bone density. As oestrogen levels drop during menopause, bone resorption (the process by which bone is broken down and its minerals released into the blood) begins to outpace bone formation, leading to a decrease in bone density. This puts postmenopausal women at a higher risk of osteoporosis and fractures.

- **Osteoporosis:** Osteoporosis is a condition characterised by weak, brittle bones that are more susceptible to fractures. Women may not be aware of bone loss until a fracture occurs, making prevention and early intervention crucial. This can be prevented with adequate vitaminD3 and K2 supplementation before menopause. Weight bearing exercise is also known to help.

- **Fracture Risk:** Common sites for fractures include the hips, spine, and wrists. These fractures can have a significant impact on quality of life, leading to reduced mobility and independence.

The Cardiovascular System: Caring for Your Heart

Cardiovascular health is another area where menopause can have a profound impact. Oestrogen helps protect the heart and blood vessels, and its decline during menopause increases the risk of cardiovascular disease (CVD).

- **Heart Disease:** Postmenopausal women are at an increased risk of developing heart disease, which includes conditions like coronary artery disease, heart attacks, and stroke. The loss of oestrogen contributes to changes in cholesterol levels, blood pressure, and the elasticity of blood vessels, all of which can increase CVD risk.

- **Cholesterol and Blood Pressure:** After menopause, levels of LDL (bad) cholesterol tend to rise, while HDL (good) cholesterol may decrease. Blood pressure may also increase, further elevating the risk of heart disease. These can be offset using omega 3 and magnesium. But always get checked before trying anything!

Mitigating the Long-Term Effects: Practical Strategies for Health

While menopause brings natural changes to your body, there are many strategies you can implement to protect your brain, bones, and cardiovascular system. By adopting a proactive approach, you can enhance your well-being and enjoy this new chapter of life with confidence and vitality.

Supporting Your Brain Health

- **Mental Stimulation:** Engage in activities that challenge your brain, such as puzzles, reading, or learning new skills. These activities can help maintain cognitive function and keep your mind sharp.

- **Regular Exercise:** Physical activity boosts blood flow to the brain, supports cognitive function, and improves mood. Aim for at least 30 minutes of moderate, weight bearing exercise most days of the week.

- **Adequate Sleep:** Prioritise good sleep hygiene to ensure restful, restorative sleep. Create a calming bedtime routine, limit caffeine and screen time before bed, and keep your bedroom cool and dark.

- **Manage Stress:** Practice stress-reducing techniques such as mindfulness meditation, yoga, or deep breathing exercises. Reducing stress can help balance mood and improve mental clarity.

Strengthening Your Bones

- **Magnesium, Calcium and Vitamin D/K:** Ensure you're getting enough magnesium, calcium and vitamin D, all of which are essential for bone health. Calcium and magnesium can be found in dairy products, leafy greens, and fortified foods, while vitamin D can be obtained through sunlight, fatty fish, mushrooms and supplements. Vitamin K can be eaten as well. Natto, a form of fermented soya, is an excellent source, as are leafy green vegetables and eggs.

- **Weight-Bearing Exercise:** Engage in weight-bearing exercises like walking, jogging, or strength training to help maintain bone density. These activities stimulate bone formation and reduce the risk of osteoporosis.

- **Bone Density Testing:** Talk to your healthcare provider about bone density testing, especially if you have risk factors for osteoporosis. Early detection allows for timely intervention to protect your bones.

- **Limit Alcohol and Quit Smoking:** Excessive alcohol consumption and smoking can accelerate bone loss. Limiting alcohol and quitting smoking are critical steps in preserving bone health.

Protecting Your Heart

- **Heart-Healthy Diet:** Adopt a diet rich in fruits, vegetables, whole grains, good quality proteins, and healthy fats, such as those found in nuts, seeds, and olive oil. This diet supports cardiovascular health and helps maintain healthy cholesterol levels.

- **Regular Physical Activity:** Exercise is a cornerstone of heart health. It helps lower blood pressure, improve cholesterol levels, and maintain a healthy weight. Aim for a combination of aerobic exercise, such as walking or swimming, and strength training.

- **Monitor Blood Pressure and Cholesterol:** Regularly check your blood pressure and cholesterol levels, and work with your healthcare provider to manage any abnormalities. Lifestyle changes and medications, if necessary, can help keep these factors in check.

- **Stress Management:** Chronic stress can negatively impact heart health. Incorporate stress-reducing practices into your daily routine to protect your cardiovascular system.

Hormone Replacement Therapy (HRT)

For some women, HRT may be a beneficial option for managing menopausal symptoms and reducing the risk of osteoporosis and heart disease. HRT involves supplementing the body with oestrogen, and sometimes progesterone, to alleviate symptoms and protect against bone loss.

- **Types of HRT:** HRT can be administered in various forms, including pills, patches, gels, and creams. Bioidentical hormones, which are chemically identical to the hormones produced by the body, are another option that some women prefer.

- **Benefits and Risks:** While HRT can provide relief from hot flashes, night sweats, and vaginal dryness, it is not without risks. These may include an increased risk of certain cancers and blood clots. It's essential to discuss the potential benefits and risks with your healthcare provider to determine if HRT is right for you. Remember that there are bioidentical options that work just as well and may have less risks, you just need to find the right healthcare provider who can properly assess you and compound what you need.

Sex after Menopause:

Yes, you can and will still have sex after menopause, but you may need additional lubrication! Thankfully these are readily available anywhere these days, so you should be able to find one suitable for your needs.

You may be more prone to urinary tract infections after menopause, so ensure your vagina keeps its acidic pH and test your microbiome to ensure that it stays healthy and keeps you healthy.

Conclusion:

Menopause is a time of change, but it's also an opportunity to focus on your health and well-being. By understanding the effects of menopause on your brain, bones, and cardiovascular system, you can take proactive steps to mitigate these changes and enjoy a fulfilling, vibrant life.

Remember, menopause is not an end, it's a new beginning. With the right strategies, support, and mindset, you can embrace this chapter with confidence, knowing that you are taking care of your body and mind in the best way possible. Reach out to your healthcare provider, lean on your support network, and prioritise your health as you navigate this transformative time.

Chapter 19

Navigating Andropause: Hormonal Changes and Strategies for Maintaining Health as Men Age

Introduction: Understanding Andropause

As men age, they undergo a series of hormonal changes that can significantly impact their health and well-being. This period, often referred to as andropause, is characterised by a gradual decline in testosterone levels, sometimes accompanied by other hormonal shifts. Unlike the more abrupt hormonal changes women experience during menopause, andropause is typically more gradual, with symptoms appearing over a span of years.

In this chapter, we will explore the physiological changes associated with andropause, the common symptoms men may experience, and the lifestyle and nutritional strategies that can help mitigate the effects of declining testosterone. Understanding andropause and taking proactive steps can help men maintain their health, energy, and vitality well into their later years.

The Hormonal Landscape of Andropause

1. **Testosterone Decline:**

   o **Overview:** Testosterone levels peak in a man's late teens to early twenties and begin to decline gradually from around the age of 30. By the time a man reaches his 50s or 60s, testosterone levels may have decreased by 1-2% per year.

   o **Impact:** This decline can affect various aspects of health, including sexual function, muscle mass, bone density, mood, and energy levels.

   o **Symptoms:** Common symptoms of low testosterone during andropause include reduced libido, erectile dysfunction, increased body fat, decreased muscle mass, fatigue, depression, and cognitive decline.

2. **Other Hormonal Changes:**

   o **DHEA and Androstenedione:** Levels of DHEA, a precursor to testosterone and oestrogen, also decline with age, potentially contributing to the symptoms of andropause.

   o **Estradiol:** As testosterone levels decline, there can be an increase in the conversion of testosterone to estradiol (a form of oestrogen), which can lead to imbalances that affect mood, energy levels, and body composition.

- o **Cortisol:** Chronic stress can lead to elevated cortisol levels, which can further exacerbate testosterone decline and contribute to symptoms like fatigue, weight gain, and mood disturbances.

Symptoms of Andropause

1. **Sexual Health:**

   - o **Reduced Libido and Erectile Dysfunction:** Lower testosterone levels can lead to a decrease in sexual desire and difficulties achieving or maintaining an erection.

   - o **Fertility Decline:** Sperm production may decrease, and the quality of sperm may decline, affecting fertility.

2. **Physical Changes:**

   - o **Muscle Loss and Increased Fat:** Testosterone is critical for maintaining muscle mass and strength. As levels decline, men may notice a loss of muscle and an increase in body fat, particularly around the abdomen.

- ○ **Bone Density:** Reduced testosterone can lead to a decrease in bone density, increasing the risk of osteoporosis and fractures.

- ○ **Hair Loss:** Hormonal changes can accelerate hair thinning and loss.

3. **Emotional and Cognitive Changes:**

   - ○ **Mood Swings and Depression:** Men may experience mood swings, irritability, and a sense of depression as testosterone levels decline.

   - ○ **Cognitive Decline:** Some men report difficulties with memory, concentration, and mental clarity during andropause.

4. **Energy Levels:**

   - ○ **Fatigue:** Persistent fatigue is a common symptom as lower testosterone levels can affect energy production and metabolism.

   - ○ **Sleep Disturbances:** Men may experience insomnia, sleep apnoea, or restless sleep, which can further contribute to feelings of fatigue.

Strategies for Maintaining Health During Andropause

1. **Exercise and Physical Activity:**

    o **Strength Training:** Regular resistance training is one of the most effective ways to combat muscle loss, improve strength, and boost testosterone levels. Aim for at least two to three sessions per week.

    o **Cardiovascular Exercise:** Incorporating aerobic activities, such as walking, running, or cycling, helps maintain cardiovascular health and supports weight management.

    o **Flexibility and Balance:** Activities like yoga, stretching, and Pilates can improve flexibility, balance, and reduce the risk of injury.

2. **Nutrition:**

    o **Healthy Fats:** Include sources of healthy fats, such as avocados, nuts, seeds, and fatty fish, to support hormone production.

    o **Protein Intake:** Adequate protein is essential for maintaining muscle mass. Incorporate lean meats, eggs, dairy, legumes, and plant-based proteins into your diet.

- ○ **Vitamins and Minerals:** Ensure adequate intake of vitamin D, zinc, and magnesium, which are crucial for testosterone production and bone health.

- ○ **Antioxidants:** Foods rich in antioxidants, such as berries, dark leafy greens, and nuts, help combat oxidative stress, which can accelerate the aging process.

3. **Stress Management:**

- ○ **Mindfulness Practices:** Meditation, deep breathing exercises, and mindfulness can help reduce stress, which is important for maintaining balanced cortisol levels and supporting testosterone production.

- ○ **Work-Life Balance:** Striking a healthy balance between work and personal life can prevent chronic stress and its negative effects on hormonal health.

- ○ **Social Connections:** Maintaining strong social connections and engaging in community activities can improve mood and reduce feelings of isolation, which are important for mental health during andropause.

4. **Sleep:**

- ○ **Sleep Hygiene:** Establishing a regular sleep routine, creating a restful environment, and avoiding stimulants like caffeine before bed can improve sleep quality.

- ○ **Addressing Sleep Disorders:** If sleep apnoea or other sleep disorders are present, seeking medical advice and appropriate treatment is essential for overall health.

5. **Hormone Replacement Therapy (HRT):**

- ○ **Testosterone Replacement:** For some men, testosterone replacement therapy (TRT) may be recommended to alleviate severe symptoms of low testosterone. It's important to work with a healthcare provider to assess the risks and benefits. If you are overweight, you run the risk of the testosterone being aromatised into oestrogen, so please ensure you are at an ideal weight before considering TRT.

- ○ **Natural Alternatives:** For those who prefer a non-pharmaceutical approach, herbal supplements such as ashwagandha, fenugreek, and tribulus terrestris may offer mild testosterone-boosting effects, not increasing testosterone overtly, but reducing the impact of stress on testosterone.

6. **Regular Health Check-Ups:**

   o **Monitoring Hormone Levels:** Regular blood tests to monitor testosterone and other hormone levels can help in managing andropause effectively.

   o **Bone Density Testing:** Periodic bone density scans may be recommended to assess the risk of osteoporosis, especially if there are other risk factors present.

   o **Cardiovascular Health:** Metabolic syndrome has a massive effect on testosterone. Regular monitoring of blood pressure, cholesterol levels, and heart health is crucial during this phase of life.

Conclusion:

Andropause is a natural part of aging, but with the right strategies, men can maintain their health, vitality, and well-being throughout this transition. By understanding the hormonal changes that occur, recognising the symptoms, and implementing lifestyle and nutritional interventions, men can navigate andropause with greater ease and continue to lead fulfilling, active lives.

Many men have successfully navigated or even reversed andropause through improving their diet, overall nutrition, muscle mass and stress responses. Unlike menopause, which is not reversible, you have much more control over the effects of andropause!

Chapter 20

Comprehensive Hormone Testing: A recap of Evaluating Thyroid, Adrenal, and Gonadal Health

Introduction: The Importance of Hormone Testing

Hormones are critical regulators of countless bodily functions, from metabolism and energy levels to reproduction and stress response. When hormone levels are imbalanced or not functioning correctly, they can lead to various health issues, such as fatigue, weight gain, mood disturbances, and infertility. Accurate hormone testing is essential for diagnosing and managing these conditions, providing a clear picture of your hormonal health.

This chapter will explore the best methods for testing thyroid, adrenal, and gonadal hormones, including the different types of samples—saliva, blood, dried blood spots, urine, and dried urine. We'll discuss what each type of test measures, how to interpret the results, and the advantages and disadvantages of each testing method.

Thyroid Hormones: Evaluating Metabolic Health

The thyroid gland plays a key role in regulating metabolism, energy production, and overall metabolic health through the secretion of thyroid hormones—primarily thyroxine (T4) and triiodothyronine (T3). Proper thyroid function is crucial for maintaining energy levels, body weight, and cognitive function.

Key Thyroid Hormones and Markers

- **Thyroid-Stimulating Hormone (TSH):** Produced by the pituitary gland, TSH signals the thyroid to produce T4 and T3. TSH is typically the first marker tested when evaluating thyroid function.

- **Free T4 (Thyroxine):** T4 is the inactive form of thyroid hormone, which is converted into the active form, T3, in the body. Free T4 measures the amount of unbound T4 available for conversion.

- **Free T3 (Triiodothyronine):** T3 is the active thyroid hormone that regulates metabolism. Free T3 measures the unbound, active form of T3 in the blood.

- **Reverse T3 (rT3):** Reverse T3 is an inactive form of T3 that can block the action of active T3 at the cellular level. High levels of rT3 may indicate a problem with T4 to T3 conversion.

- **Thyroid Antibodies:** Antibodies such as anti-thyroperoxidase (TPO) and anti-thyroglobulin (TgAb) indicate autoimmune thyroid conditions like Hashimoto's thyroiditis and Graves' disease.

Testing Methods for Thyroid Hormones

- **Blood Tests (Serum):** Blood tests are the most common method for measuring thyroid hormones. A simple blood draw can provide levels of TSH, free T4, free T3, rT3, and thyroid antibodies. Blood tests are highly accurate and provide a comprehensive picture of thyroid function. However, they reflect only a snapshot of hormone levels at the time of the test.

Advantages: Accurate, comprehensive, widely available.

Disadvantages: Reflects hormone levels at a single point in time, may miss fluctuations throughout the day.

- **Dried Blood Spot (DBS):** Dried blood spot testing involves collecting a small sample of blood from a finger prick onto a special card. Once dried, the card is sent to a lab for analysis. DBS can measure TSH, free T4, and free T3 as well as antibodies and is convenient for at-home testing. You can also assess the nutrients and toxins that affect thyroid health using the same DBS card with some labs.

Advantages: Convenient, less invasive, suitable for at-home testing.

Disadvantages: Limited availability of tests.

Adrenal Hormones: Assessing the Stress Response

The adrenal glands produce hormones essential for stress response, metabolism, and electrolyte balance, including cortisol, cortisone and DHEA (dehydroepiandrosterone). Proper adrenal function is vital for coping with stress, maintaining energy levels, and regulating blood pressure.

Key Adrenal Hormones and Markers

- **Cortisol/cortisone:** The primary stress hormone, cortisol is released in response to stress and follows a diurnal rhythm, peaking in the morning and declining throughout the day. It helps regulate metabolism, blood sugar, and inflammation. It can be converted into cortisone if needed. Cortisone is the inactive form of cortisol.

- **DHEA:** A precursor to sex hormones, DHEA is produced by the adrenal glands and helps buffer the effects of cortisol. It also plays a role in immune function and aging.

Testing Methods for Adrenal Hormones

- **Saliva Tests:** Saliva testing is a common method for measuring cortisol and DHEA levels. Multiple samples are collected throughout the day to assess the diurnal pattern of cortisol. Saliva testing is non-invasive and reflects the free, active form of the hormone.

Advantages: Non-invasive, easy to collect multiple samples, reflects active hormone levels.

Disadvantages: Limited to certain hormones, may be affected by saliva production or contamination.

- **Blood Tests (Serum):** Blood tests can measure cortisol and DHEA levels. However, a single blood draw may not accurately reflect the diurnal pattern of cortisol.

Advantages: Accurate for certain hormones and widely available.

Disadvantages: Invasive, may not capture diurnal cortisol patterns.

- **Dried Urine Tests:** Dried urine testing, provides a comprehensive assessment of adrenal hormones, including cortisol, cortisone (inactive form of cortisol), DHEA, and their metabolites. It offers insights into both the levels and the metabolism of these hormones.

Advantages: Comprehensive, provides both hormone levels and metabolites, convenient for at-home testing.

Disadvantages: Limited availability, more expensive than other tests.

- **24-Hour Urine Tests:** This method involves collecting all urine produced over 24 hours to measure cortisol, DHEA, and other adrenal hormones. It provides a total output rather than a snapshot, offering a comprehensive view of hormone production.

Advantages: Comprehensive, reflects total hormone output over 24 hours.

Disadvantages: Inconvenient, may miss fluctuations in hormone levels.

Gonadal Hormones: Understanding Reproductive Health

Gonadal hormones, including oestrogen, progesterone, and testosterone, play essential roles in reproductive health, sexual function, and overall well-being. Imbalances in these hormones can lead to menstrual irregularities, infertility, low libido, and other health issues.

Key Gonadal Hormones and Markers

- **Oestrogen (Estradiol, Estrone, Estriol):** Oestrogen is critical for reproductive health, bone density, and cardiovascular function. Estradiol (E2) is the most potent form of oestrogen, while estrone (E1) and estriol (E3) also play important roles.

- **Progesterone:** Produced primarily during the luteal phase of the menstrual cycle and in pregnancy, progesterone prepares the uterus for implantation and supports early pregnancy. It also balances the effects of oestrogen.

- **Testosterone:** While often associated with male health, testosterone is also important for women, influencing libido, bone density, and muscle mass.

- **Sex Hormone Binding Globulin (SHBG):** SHBG is a protein that binds to sex hormones, particularly testosterone and oestrogen, regulating their availability and activity in the body.

Testing Methods for Gonadal Hormones

- **Blood Tests (Serum):** Blood tests are the standard method for measuring gonadal hormones, including estradiol, progesterone, testosterone, LH/FSH and SHBG. Blood tests can provide accurate measurements of total and free hormone levels, but they reflect only a single point in time.

Advantages: Accurate, widely available, provides both total and free hormone levels.

Disadvantages: Reflects hormone levels at a single point in time, may miss fluctuations throughout the cycle.

- **Saliva Tests:** Saliva testing can be used to measure free, active levels of oestrogen, progesterone, and testosterone. It is often used for assessing hormone fluctuations throughout the menstrual cycle.

Advantages: Non-invasive, reflects free hormone levels, suitable for multiple time-point testing.

Disadvantages: Limited availability of certain tests, may be affected by saliva production.

- **Dried Urine Tests:** Dried urine tests provide a comprehensive analysis of gonadal hormones, including their metabolites. This method offers insights into both the levels and metabolism of oestrogen, progesterone, and testosterone.

Advantages: Comprehensive, reflects both hormone levels and metabolism, convenient for at-home testing.

Disadvantages: Limited availability, more expensive than other tests.

- **Dried Blood Spot (DBS):** Dried blood spot testing can measure estradiol, progesterone, and testosterone levels. It is convenient for at-home testing and provides accurate measurements, particularly for monitoring hormone replacement therapy (HRT).

Advantages: Convenient, less invasive, suitable for at-home testing.

Disadvantages: Limited availability, may not provide as detailed information as serum tests.

- **24-Hour Urine Tests:** Like adrenal hormone testing, 24-hour urine tests can be used to measure oestrogen, progesterone, and testosterone levels, offering a comprehensive view of hormone production over an entire day.

Advantages: Comprehensive, reflects total hormone output over 24 hours.

Disadvantages: Inconvenient, may miss fluctuations in hormone levels.

Conclusion:

Hormone testing is a critical tool in assessing and managing thyroid, adrenal, and gonadal health. The choice of testing method depends on the specific hormones being evaluated, the patient's symptoms, and the clinical context. Understanding the strengths and limitations of each testing

Chapter 21

Real life stories, some of them in their own words, the rest from the perspective of the practice.

Patient A - (39 year old female) Multiple failed IVF/miscarriages – her story in her words:

16 September 2021: I started IVF in Feb 2020. I had 1 frozen transfer which didn't work, so the next month another one, which resulted in a pregnancy to 12 weeks (missed miscarriage resulting in a hospital stay due to loss of blood).

I then had another frozen transfer in august 2020, which didn't work, so in October a full fresh IVF cycle whereupon I was pregnant for 16 weeks. at 16 weeks (feb 2021), my waters randomly broke and I had to deliver the baby as well as getting fungal sepsis and a bacterial infection. I needed a month off work and 2 weeks of intravenous drugs as well as 4 nights in hospital.

I had another round of ivf in April 2021 but the doctors recommended freezing the embryos as I was still testing positive for group b strep and candida kefir in swabs, both of which should have been eradicated from the medication I had had. I have had another course of antibiotics since but it didn't appear to have helped the group b strep. The candida kefyr last tested negative following 2 courses of dequalinium chloride pessaries, but I had been told it was likely to come back if I went on antibiotics for the group b strep again.

I also had covid in early august and have had a cough for 4 months. My husband had also lost work during the pandemic so there were financial stressors. He was not wanting to wait to go through another IVF cycle, so there is pressure from his side to undergo another cycle, which I was in, during my first consultation with Dr Shania.

I had no symptoms but psychologically I have found things hard. the hospital carried out every test they could on me and the baby and did not find any issues apart from as above. At this point I am suffering migraines and frequent headaches; I have acne and salt cravings. My periods are very irregular and heavy, and I have PMS.

The approach:

As patient A was in her next IVF cycle, there was not much that could be done as she was having her eggs extracted the following week. She was told to come back if it didn't work and to allow 3 months to test and correct what was found. She was put her on the Reset plan while we waited for her test results to come back.

She came back when that IVF cycle failed and did a DNA test centred around the genes that ensure a healthy pregnancy, along with a. dried urine test for hormones and a gut test. When she came back for her results review, her headaches and skin had already improved. Her medical symptom questionnaire results had improved from 42 to 16 (the lower the better).

She was prescribed a program based on her results, in her DNA, methylation was a high priority. In her dried urine, she had very low oestrogen and in her gut test, she had minor imbalances.

She was given a formula for stress, some probiotics specific to her needs. A formula that helps oestrogen production and then a good prenatal supplement that covered methylation. She was also advised to use oestrogen during her next pregnancy.

Her next embryo took and resulted in a healthy baby boy, born almost exactly a year from when she first started the program. If we didn't pick up her low oestrogen (which was never tested while going through her IVF) this may not have had the same result!

Patient B – (60 year old female) – Post menopausal vaginal pain, her story.

When I met patient C, she was generally well, post menopausal and cheerful, however, she had been suffering for pain in her vagina for a few years which was preventing her from entering into a sexual relationship. She has been prescribed vaginal oestrogen but that hadn't solved the issue. She really didn't seem to have any other issues, but the pain was reported as severe and constant!

We ran a vaginal microbiome test and she had low diversity and none of the acid producing bacteria that would lower the pH of the vagina to a healthy 4.5. Her pH was almost alkaline, which isn't healthy.

She also had high risk for developing vaginal bacteriosis (VB) a common condition that often causes smelly vaginal discharge, but isn't generally associated with the pain she was describing.

I prescribed an over-the-counter vaginal pessary for VB along with an oral and vaginal probiotic that contained Lactobacillus crispatus LCR01 (DSM 24619), Lactobacillus fermentum LF10 (DSM 19187), Lactobacillus acidophilus LA02 (DSM 21712).

We retested after a month. At this point she was pain free and in a new, sexually active relationship!

Her follow up results showed she needed to stay on the probiotics to maintain the new microbiome, but her pH had lowered into the normal range and most importantly, she was pain free.

Patient C – (42 year old female) - sudden onset of menstrual changes, heavy bleeding, her story in her own words.

May 2018, I had never had menstrual irregularities, in fact, I had a "normal" cycle, until I moved house, which had a damp issue. Within a few months of moving into this house, my cycle became so heavy and full of massive clots. It came out of nowhere and was so heavy that I was changing a night pad, every hour! I also started to gain weight.

I did a dried urine test and it showed very high oestrogen, with high levels of the 4OH metabolite, also known as The Bad metabolite and high levels of cortisol. I also opted to test for mycotoxins as it was suspected that there was mold in the damp. I tested positive for zearanolone.

I also went for an ultrasound and was diagnosed with fibroids. The doctor wanted to prescribe the Mirena but `I have never done well on hormones so opted to support my adrenals and detoxification processes.

My stress levels improved and so did the symptoms. I had a normal cycle for the next 18 months, but then my stress was triggered, severely, and the symptoms returned. I opted to treat the fibroids with uterine artery embolization, and this improved the symptoms immediately. I did however continue to monitor my hormones as I was made aware by this experience that even though I may have treated the fibroids, the oestrogen detoxification and stress issues were still potentially there. I continue on my program and report that I am healthy, fit and energetic.

I am on a program designed around my genetics and my regular hormone checks and includes adrenal support, oestrogen specific support, along with nutrients that my body has a higher need for, such a b vitamins and omega 3. While I take my supplements diligently, I also support myself through a healthy diet and regular exercise.

I am grateful for the tests as I would have been high risk for many health conditions that are now being prevented.

I am approaching perimenopause, but still have a regular cycle with no symptoms yet, I am hoping that with the continued guidance of this book, that I will be able to transition gently into my next chapter.

Patient D – (46 year old male) - erectile dysfunction and low libido, in his words

Generally, I feel pretty well! I eat healthily, no smoking or drinking. Generally content.

Some stress from financial insecurity, tax credits, not having a stable home (staying with friends). Currently a little isolated due to rural location.

Childhood: stable, safe and conventional. Developed asthma and eczema early in life. Use of steroids and antibiotics typical in childhood but no major injuries/illnesses. Lot of sugar, convenience food and microwave/oven dinners. SEX Long standing lack of confidence with sex. Little sexual education and verbal bullying around body shape/penis size when young at school. No support to talk about the issue when young...felt very alone and anxious with it. Inability to form relationships with women. Lost virginity when 21, little sex before 30. Never been in a long term relationship.

Some sexual partners I have been able to get an erection and others not. Never been able to have 'normal sex' for sustained periods. Inability to achieve erections or when I do, it's not very solid and will easily wane. Little experience with penetration, so often feel anxious and want to orgasm quickly...premature ejaculation.

Have had tests at GP ten years ago around these issues...not sure exactly what they tested for but normal stuff. Came back reading normal levels. Have done explorations into personal development, anger/grief release around the bullying, breathwork, tantra, homeopathy etc around the issue but haven't found an answer.

Have occasionally used Viagra on and off for about 15 years with some success. Side effects: headaches. Used Viagra earlier this year a number of times with a new partner. Not together now. In last few months I have noticed something changing in my body and ability to achieve any kind of erection. Something feels even more relaxed and softened. It felt time for another round of tests.

The approach:

We ran a dried urine and full blood panel. Not surprisingly his adrenals were flagged in both results and his testosterone was very low in the dried urine (low end of normal in blood).

My clinic doesn't prescribe hormones, but I work with clinics that do, so he was referred to one of my associated clinics as he wanted to try testosterone therapy while treating his adrenals.

Patient E – (51 year old female) – early menopause in her mid 30's

When I met patient E she had already been post menopausal for 15 years. She had been an alcoholic and believed that was what caused her early menopause. She was on HRT but was experiencing severe anxiety and brain fog as well as bloating and general inflammation. She had tried various diets but had not resolved her symptoms.

We did a thorough history, including questions about her possible exposure to mould and her overall gut health. She mentioned her home had experienced water damage.

We did a variety of gut tests on her, including one for SIBO (small intestinal bacterial overgrowth) which was positive. We also assessed her adrenals. But she was hesitant to test for mycotoxins, which we believed were the cause of most if not all her symptoms, including the SIBO!

She was treated for the SIBO, but as a precaution, was also treated for mould. This includes getting air purifiers and infra red sweating. We added a herbal adrenal formula and detox support.

We are happy to report, that she is healthy and feeling much better! The bloating has gone and she is motivated to investigate the mycotoxins but even without testing for them, that fact that she improved very quickly on the right program, seems to confirm that mould was indeed the main culprit, even though her hormones were being blamed for the symptoms!

Her story serves to remind people that treating the gut and root cause is the key to chronic cases resolving.

Patient F – (35 year old female) – extreme allergies and mood disorders, bad reaction to HRT

Patient F started to experience the symptoms of perimenopause and consulted her doctor who prescribed oestrogen as HRT. She had never been allergic to anything, but suffered a few distressing anaphylactic episodes that resulted in hospitalisation.

On examination of her hormones, it showed that although she had some symptoms of perimenopause, that she was oestrogen dominant and progesterone deficient.

She was advised that progesterone may be what she needs and was referred to a prescriber. She went on a program to support oestrogen detoxification and histamine binding and that, along with the progesterone, has improved dramatically,

This story serves to demonstrate, that testing is important during perimenopause as there are the potentials to be oestrogen dominant before the oestrogen decreases and HRT is required. She continues to test her hormones and when needed, will add bio identical oestrogen by her prescriber.

She is doing well on her program and has not had any anaphylaxis since being on it.

Laboratories that can assist you with testing:

If you struggle to find a lab that will do the testing, please go to the contact page on wwww.drshania.com and someone will be able to assist you.

Alletess - https://foodallergy.com/ - do the IGE, IGG, and IGA test called the Expanded mould panel

Analytical Research Labs (ARL) - https://arltma.com/ does hair analysis

Diagnostic solutions lab

- https://www.diagnosticsolutionslab.com/ do the microbiome analysis and organic acid tests

Doctors Data Inc - https://www.doctorsdata.com/ do a number of tests, including hair analysis and hormones.

Genova - https://www.gdx.net/ and https://www.gdx.net/uk/ do a number of useful tests, including organic acids

Gut ID - https://www.gutid.com/ for microbiome assessment

Envirobiomics - https://www.envirobiomics.com/ test moulds and co-infections

KBMO - https://kbmodiagnostics.co.uk or https://kbmodiagnostics.com test for food sensitivities

Mosaic DX - https://mosaicdx.com/ do the Mycotox and Organic acids tests

Precision analytical - https://dutchtest.com/ test hormones

Real-time labs - https://realtimelab.com/ test mycotoxins and environmental toxicants

Trace Elements Inc. - https://www.traceelements.com/ and https://www.mineralcheck.com/ do hair analysis

Vibrant Wellness - https://www.vibrant-wellness.com/ toxins and gut testing

ZRT - https://www.zrtlab.com/ test blood metals as well as hormones

An excellent resource for finding a practitioner:

https://www.ifm.org/find-a-practitioner/

Visual contrast sensitivity test:

https://www.vcstest.com/

Environmental testing and rehabilitation:

Pure maintenance - they are in the UK and USA https://www.puremaintenanceuk.com/

Mould lab - https://mouldlab.co.uk/

Eurofins USA and Canada - https://www.emlab.com/

Gupta program:

https://guptaprogram.com/aff/909/

Sourcing good supplements

If you struggle to find supplements and you are in the UK, USA, EU or RSA, please go to the contact page on wwww.drshania.com and someone will be able to assist you.

I use and recommend the following brands, but there are other excellent brands that your practitioner may advise instead:

- Allergy Research
- Designs for Health
- Metagenics, Nutri advanced, Amipro
- Researched Nutritional's
- Xymogen
- Pure encapsulations
- NOW
- Dr's Best
- Microbiome Labs
- Thorne

But there are many more and you should use whatever your healthcare provider recommends.

Continue your health journey by scanning the QR code

www.ingramcontent.com/pod-product-compliance
Lightning Source LLC
Chambersburg PA
CBHW052014030426
42335CB00026B/3147